# Empowering Patients: How to Understand Drug Quality Information

Saniya

## Table of Contents

# 1. Introduction

According to the German Medicinal Products Act (Arzneimittelgesetz), the quality of a drug is defined as "[...] *the nature of a medicinal product, determined by identity, content, purity and other chemical, physical and biological properties or by the manufacturing procedure*" [1]. The quality of a certain pharmaceutical product is ensured by its compendial monograph, which includes tests for its identity, purity and content. At the global level, the pharmaceutical quality assessment based on Good Manufacturing Practice (GMP) is regulated by the Quality Guidelines of the International Conference on Harmonization of Technical Requirements for Registration of Pharmaceuticals for Human Use (ICH) [2].

In the European Pharmacopoeia (Ph.Eur.), the purity of a drug is examined, among others, by the test for related substances, where the amount of impurities should not exceed certain limits [3]. The determination of the purity of a pharmaceutical product is a challenging issue, because the impurity profile depends on the production process [4,5]. For example, a change in the synthesis route of a compound may change its impurity profile, as reported on the "valsartan affair" in 2018, where the replacement of a reaction solvent and a reagent within the manufacturing pathway led to the formation of toxic nitrosamines in different sartan drugs [6,7]. Consequently, limits for $N$-nitrosodimethylamine (NDMA) and $N$-nitrosodiethylamine (NDEA) were established in the respective monograph of the Ph.Eur. [8]. However, a suitable test for those impurities is currently in the process of implementation. Another example of insufficient drug quality was reported within the frame of the heparin contamination crisis in early 2008, where unfractioned heparin was intentionally contaminated with oversulfated chondroitin sulfate (OSCS), causing anaphylactiod reactions [9,10]. Therefore, former compendial monographs had to be revised to implement suitable tests to evaluate the amount of OSCS [11]. These exemplified incidents clearly demonstrate the urgent need of thorough quality control and assurance, which are key factors to ensure drug safety.

To cope with the challenges in quality assessment of pharmaceutical products, many types of analytical techniques are available [12]. Every technique has its advantages and drawbacks, which makes appropriate quality assessment a tailor made issue. Amongst the various analytical tools available, high performance liquid chromatography (HPLC), capillary electrophoresis (CE) and nuclear magnetic resonance (NMR) spectroscopy were applied in this work to evaluate the impurities and degradation products of pharmaceutical compounds and will be briefly described in the following.

## 1.1  High performance liquid chromatography

Chromatographic separation techniques are based on distribution and adsorption processes of the analytes between a stationary and a mobile phase, which carries the analytes towards the detector [13]. Separation of analytes is achieved by adjusting the properties of both phases. In HPLC, many different stationary phases are available to cover various separation modes, e.g. reversed phase (RP) or ion-pairing (IP) chromatography [14,15]. Stationary phases are usually based on chemically modified silica and provide different chemical properties related to the chemical modification [16]. As a rule of thumb, the polarity of the stationary phase should be similar to that of the analyte. Hence, for the separation of hydrophilic analytes, hydrophilic stationary phases are preferably used, which consist, for example, of unmodified silica or polar modifications like cyano-, diol-, amine- or amide groups. For hydrophobic compounds, rather hydrophobic silica modifications are employed, e.g. long alkyl chains (e.g. C-4, C-8, C-18) or phenyl groups. Currently, most of the separations which are performed by means of HPLC are carried out using RP columns; in fact, for the determination of related substances in the Ph.Eur., the predominant method is RP-LC [14,16].

Some stationary phases are "endcapped", which means that residues of unmodified, active silica are treated with methyltrichlorosilane to further decrease the polarity and reduce peak tailing of basic analytes by secondary interactions. Other stationary phases consist of sulfonate or quaternary amine groups, acting as ion exchangers. In mixed-mode stationary phases, different types of separation mechanisms and, thus, chemical properties are combined. For enantioseparation, chiral stationary phases are available, which are composed of e.g. polysaccharides or proteins [15].

Apart from chemical properties, further characteristics like length and diameter of the column, carbon loading, particle size and porosity are likely to affect the chromatographic result and have to be considered during method development.

The choice of the mobile phase usually depends on the stationary phase employed and is crucial for optimal separation of the analytes. Some important factors that have to be considered include the elution strength, pH value, and compatibility with the detector (e.g. UV-cutoff, volatility). Typical mobile phases for RP-HPLC are mixtures of water and organic solvents, with or without additives like buffer salts or ion-pairing reagents [16]. The composition of the mobile phase can be kept constant (isocratic elution) or varied during the measurement to improve separation efficiency (gradient elution).

Various detectors are available to cope with the versatility of analytes and analytical issues. UV/Vis detectors are frequently used for molecules with a chromophore; for non-chromophore compounds, aerosol-based detectors such as the charged aerosol detector (CAD) may be employed [17]. The application of a mass spectrometer (MS) additionally offers the possibility of structure elucidation of unknown analytes. Modern MS instruments provide outstanding sensitivity and selectivity, but purchase and maintenance are usually quite expensive.

Combining simplicity, variability, high robustness and precision, HPLC is one of the most important separation techniques in pharmaceutical analysis, as it is shown by numerous assay methods and tests on related substances in compendial monographs [18-20].

## 1.2 Capillary electrophoresis

In CE, analytes are separated due to different migration velocities inside a capillary under the influence of an electrical field [21]. Detection is commonly based on UV/Vis or fluorescence spectroscopy and takes place inside the capillary. However, in contrast to HPLC, analytes are migrating through the detection window with different velocities, thus the migration time corrected peak area has to be used for calculation. Fused silica capillaries filled with buffer as background electrolyte (BGE) or gel in capillary gel electrophoresis (CGE) are usually employed for separation. The inner surface of an untreated fused silica capillary consists of silanol groups which influence the electroosmotic flow (EOF) due to their degree of dissociation ($pK_a \approx 5$ [22,23]). Migration velocities and thus separation efficiency of various analytes can be modified by modulating the capillary's inner surface [24,25]. Several BGE additives can be used to extend the applicability of CE. For example, in micellar electrokinetic chromatography (MEKC), surfactants such as sodium dodecyl sulfate (SDS) are added to act as pseudo-stationary phases by the formation of micelles, which interact with the analytes depending on their lipophilicity [26]. Large (poly)cationic compounds such as ionic liquids are reported to modulate the EOF to improve separation of analytes with similar electrophoretic mobilities [27]. One of the most considerable applications of CE is the separation of chiral compounds by adding chiral selectors (CS) to the BGE [28,29], which will be discussed in more detail in section 1.4.

Severe drawbacks of CE are its comparatively low robustness and sensitivity; the latter is due to the narrow capillaries used (Fig. 1) and hence the short optical path lengths (usually 25 - 150 µm internal diameter). Several techniques for sensitivity improvement are available to overcome this problem, including capillary diameter enlargements, off- and on-line sample treatment and in-capillary sample preconcentration [30,31]. Although several applications of CE in pharmaceutical analysis have been reported [32,33], it is still sparingly implemented in the Ph.Eur. However, due to its advantages of high method versatility, separation efficiency and speed, low sample and solvent consumption and costs, CE has become a widely used technique for the separation of analytically challenging enantiomers [34] and biological macromolecules like proteins, sugars or DNA [35].

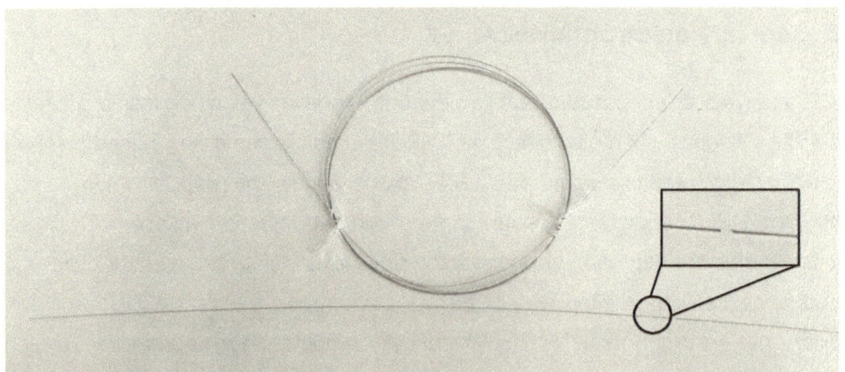

**Figure 1.** Fused silica capillary (BGB Analytik, 363 µm OD, 75 µm ID) employed in CE, shown wound up (top) and cut to 50 cm length (bottom). The capillaries are covered with a polyimide layer to improve flexibility and handling. The detection window (shown enlarged) was created by carefully burning away the polyimide layer at this place. Photo was taken by the author.

## 1.3 Nuclear magnetic resonance spectroscopy

In contrast to HPLC and CE, NMR spectroscopy is not a separation technique. Here, atom nuclei with a magnetic momentum, such as $^1$H, $^{13}$C, $^{15}$N or $^{31}$P, are irradiated with a radio frequency source in a static magnetic field. If the irradiation frequency meets the resonance frequency of the nucleus (the so called Larmor frequency), excitation and subsequent relaxation give rise to a signal in the Fourier transformed spectrum [36]. Nuclear resonances and signal patterns are highly dependent on their chemical environment within the analyte, which makes one- and multidimensional NMR spectroscopy an excellent tool for structure elucidation in organic synthesis and drug development, especially when combined with mass spectral information. Thus, it is a widely employed technique to identify drugs and their impurities [37].

Besides structure elucidation, NMR spectroscopy is suitable for quantification purposes (qNMR). The signal intensity is directly proportional to the nuclei giving rise to the respective signal, which determines NMR spectroscopy to be a primary method according to the committee for chemical measurements (Comité Consultatif pour la Quantité de Matière, CCQM) [38-40]. For quantification, mostly $^1$H nuclei are used because of their relatively high natural abundance in the magnitude of organic molecules (about 99.99%), which is not the case for $^{13}$C nuclei (about 1.07%). Therefore, analytes are usually dissolved in deuterated solvents. Quantification in NMR spectroscopy can be performed in various ways [41-44], including the pulse length based concentration determination (PULCON) [45-47] or the Electronic Reference To access *In vivo* Concentrations (ERETIC) methodology [48,49]. Furthermore, the residual solvent signal [50,51] or its $^{13}$C satellites [52] can be used as special kinds of internal standards. Even though sensitivity of NMR spectroscopy is comparably low, it can be easily enhanced by e.g. increasing the number of scans, which, however, leads to longer analysis times.

Numerous applications of (q)NMR in drug analysis were reported [53,54]. In the Ph.Eur., NMR spectroscopy is used for identification purposes, e.g. peptides [55] and heparins [56-58], but also for the determination of compositions of polymers like macrogols [59]. However, even though NMR spectroscopy is a very powerful tool in pharmaceutical analysis, it is still sparingly implemented in the Ph.Eur.

## 1.4 Analytical techniques for chiral recognition

Two enantiomers of a chiral compound are the nonsuperimposable image and mirror image of each other. Since their physicochemical properties are identical, special analytical approaches are required for separation.

One strategy for enantioseparation is the indirect method which is based on the reaction of the chiral analyte with an enantiomerically pure reagent, forming a pair of diastereomers. Due to the differences in their physicochemical properties, the diastereomers can be separately analyzed by means of common achiral methodologies. Many chiral derivatizing reagents (CDR) are available to cover a wide range of analytes [15]. However, a complication of the derivatization method is the requirement of highly pure and stable CDRs to avoid the formation of more than one pair of diastereomers. Furthermore, the reaction between CDR and analyte should be selective with respect to other functional groups that could undergo derivatization. The indirect method is especially used in NMR spectroscopy for the determination of the enantiomeric purity and absolute configuration of enantiomers. Here, the mostly used CDR is α-methoxy-α-(trifluoromethyl)phenylacetic acid (MTPA), also known as Mosher's reagent [60].

Another approach to chiral recognition is the direct method, involving the formation of non-covalent diasteromeric complexes between the chiral analyte and a chiral selector (CS) [15]. Apart from the Mosher's method, chiral recognition in NMR spectroscopy is provided using chiral lanthanide shift reagents (LSR) or chiral solvating agents (CSA) [60]. LSRs are organic multi-coordinated complexes containing a lanthanide metal such as europium or ytterbium, forming addition complexes with the chiral analyte. However, LSRs cause paramagnetic line broadening which gets more significant with higher magnetic field strengths, resulting in decreased resolution [61,62]. Hence, chiral LSRs are mostly replaced by organic CSAs, which cover chemical entities like cyclodextrins (CD), crown ethers, α-methoxyphenylacetic acids or chiral polypeptide liquid crystals [62].

In chromatographic separation techniques, the CS can be either added to the mobile phase (chiral mobile phase additive, CMPA) or connected to the chromatographic support, forming a chiral stationary phase (CSP). The practical approach using CMPAs is limited due to several drawbacks (e.g. low robustness, incompatibility with detector), whereas the CSPs are predominantly employed because of their straightforwardness and convenience [15,63,64]. A large number of CSPs are available, which are based on e.g. polysaccharides, macrocyclic antibiotics, or peptides, to cope with various analytes [63]. However, most of those stationary phases are not very stable and rather expensive.

In chiral CE, the CS is added to the BGE, causing diastereomeric interactions with the analyte isomers according to the host-guest principle [26,65]. The most widely used CSs are CDs, which are usually composed of 6, 7 or 8 glucose monomers ($\alpha$-, $\beta$-, and $\gamma$-CD, respectively), forming a circular, cone like structure with a hydrophobic inner and a hydrophilic outer environment. Apart from native CDs, various derivatives and CD mixtures are employed to improve selectivity [66]. Besides CDs, numerous other substances such as crown ethers, antibiotics, proteins or chiral ionic liquids have been reported to act as CSs as well [28,67]. Similar to the CSPs in chromatographic techniques, the capillary's inner surface can be modified with a CS, e.g. heparin [68].

## 1.5 Impurities in substances for pharmaceutical use

Comprehensive knowledge of (potential toxic) impurities of a drug is crucial to assure safety. Impurities may be drug-related or non-drug-related, and their presence and formation depends on many factors.

### 1.5.1 Pharmaceuticals from natural sources

Approximately 25 - 50% of the marketed drugs originate from natural sources [69]. Pharmaceutical substances like several alkaloids, antibiotics and excipients are obtained by isolating them from their matrices and related compounds followed by purification [70]. Natural sources for pharmaceuticals are multifarious (e.g. animals, plants, fungi), and the matrices are often complex component mixtures, contributing to the impurity profile of the isolate. For instance, morphine is isolated from crude opium, which contains many structurally related alkaloids. Due to the incomplete isolation process, they may potentially occur in the final drug product and have to be considered for quality assurance [71].

Apart from the matrix, the drug or excipient itself may consist of multiple components. For example, paraffins are mixtures of structurally different mineral oil hydrocarbons

(MOH), which are generally categorized as mineral oil saturated hydrocarbons (MOSH) and mineral oil aromatic hydrocarbons (MOAH) [72]. Despite various refining, extraction and purification steps, potential carcinogenic MOAH (especially the polycyclic aromatic hydrocarbons, PAH) can reside within the final paraffin product and are thus limited by a compendial test [73-77].

### 1.5.2 Synthetic pharmaceuticals

For chemically synthesized active pharmaceutical ingredients (API), the ICH guideline Q3A(R2) classifies impurities into three categories: organic and inorganic impurities and residual solvents, which mainly originate from manufacturing procedure or storage [78]. Therefore, all chemicals used within the synthesis pathway may be found in the final product, e.g. unreacted starting materials, catalysts and solvents. Of note, it must be taken into account that all chemicals and materials employed within the manufacturing procedure may contain impurities as well. Furthermore, impurities produced during synthesis, such as intermediates and by-products, including undesired chiral isomers in enantioselective synthesis, have to be considered [79]. As outlined, the impurity profile of a chemically synthesized drug is highly affected by the synthesis process and can therefore be controlled and predicted to some extent.

### 1.5.3 Degradation products

Due to manufacturing, storage and aging, degradation products of APIs are commonly found impurities. The ICH guidelines Q1A(R2) [80] and Q1B [81] cover the (photo)stability testing of new drug substances and products, Q5C [82] describes the stability testing of biological/biotechnological products. Stability-indicating investigations are performed under certain environmental conditions (Tab. 1) to evaluate the degradation pathways and profiles or changes in biological activity of the API.

**Table 1.** Storage conditions and length of stability-indicating studies for new drug substances and products according to ICH Q1A(R2) [80]. RH: relative humidity.

| Study | Storage condition | Minimum time period covered by data at submission |
|---|---|---|
| Long term* | 25 ± 2 °C / 60% ± 5% RH or 30 ± 2 °C / 65% ± 5% RH | 12 months |
| Intermediate** | 30 ± 2 °C / 65% ± 5% RH | 6 months |
| Accelerated | 40 ± 2 °C / 75% ± 5% RH | 6 months |

*It is up to the applicant to decide whether long term stability studies are performed at 25 ± 2 °C / 60% ± 5% RH or 30 ± 2 °C / 65% ± 5% RH.

**If 30 ± 2 °C / 65% ± 5% RH is the long-term condition, there is no intermediate condition.

Formation of degradation products is due to the chemical instability of the API molecule, which is caused by several mechanisms, e.g. hydrolysis (especially esters and amides), (aut)oxidation, decarboxylation, photolysis, thermolysis, isomerization, polymerization or Maillard reaction [79,83]. One must keep in mind that excipients may promote degradation processes of the API in the final drug product [84]. Similar to the synthetic process, knowledge about the chemical behavior of the API facilitates the prediction of potentially formed degradation products.

Forced degradation studies (stress tests) are performed under more severe conditions than the stability tests described by the ICH guideline Q1A(R2) and aim to support the identification of degradation products and evaluation of degradation pathways [80]. However, the guideline does not provide detailed information about the experimental conditions or practical approaches. Therefore, several suggestions were made on the implementation of stress tests [85]. The mostly used conditions for forced degradation studies are summarized in Tab. 2.

**Table 2.** Conditions mostly used for forced degradation studies as described in [85]. N.A.: not applicable; RH: relative humidity.

| Degradation type | Experimental conditions | Storage conditions | Sampling time (days) |
| --- | --- | --- | --- |
| Hydrolysis | 0.1 M HCl | 40 °C, 60 °C | |
| | 0.1 M NaOH | 40 °C, 60 °C | |
| Oxidation | 3% $H_2O_2$ | 25 °C, 60 °C | |
| Photolytic | Light 1 x ICH* | N.A. | 1,3,5 |
| | Light 3 x ICH | | |
| Thermal | Heat chamber | 60 °C | |
| | | 60 °C / 75% RH | |
| | | 80 °C | |
| | | 80 °C / 75% RH | |

*1 x ICH ≙ illumination of 1.2 million lux hours.

## 1.6 Principal Component Analysis

In recent years, for handling large amounts of data, chemometric techniques have become a valuable tool. Data, which is generated from spectrometers for instance, usually contain numerous variables (multivariate data), which can be condensed to extract the relevant information [86]. A comprehensive toolbox of multivariate data analysis methods is available to deal with various analytical questions. In the Ph.Eur., an introduction to a selection of chemometric techniques is given to provide information for good chemometric practices and requirements [87].

Explorative, unsupervised techniques like the principal component analysis (PCA) are usually the first approach in chemometric processing. The main variance within the dataset is visualized by decomposing the variables of the original data into few correlated latent variables, the principal components [87]. As a result, a simplified overview of the main characteristics of the data is obtained, which enables the detection of similarities, patterns or groupings among objects and relationships between objects and variables [86,88]. The clusters can be further investigated using e.g. hierarchical cluster analysis (HCA). Supervised multivariate regression methods, such as partial least square (PLS) regression, are applied to evaluate the functional relationship between a measured and a target value, which is usually hard to measure directly, e.g. quality characteristics. A prediction model can be applied to determine the target value of unknown samples after calibration and validation steps [86].

Meanwhile, multivariate data analysis is an inherent application in the quality control of drug products. In combination with techniques like NMR, (near) infrared (N)IR, or Raman spectroscopy, authenticity of drugs and herbal medicines can be checked and drug manufacturing processes can be controlled and optimized as part of the process analytical technology (PAT) [89-91].

## 1.7 References

[1] Medicinal Products Act (Arzneimittelgesetz – AMG), Medicinal Products Act in the version published on 12 December 2005 (Federal Law Gazette [BGBl.]) Part I p. 3394, last amended by Article 11 of the Act of 6 May 2019 (Federal Law Gazette I p. 646), Section 4 sentence 15. Available from: https://www.gesetze-im-internet.de/englisch_amg/englisch_amg.html#p0092. Accessed October 23th 2020.

[2] International Council for Harmonization, Quality Guidelines.

[3] EDQM, Strasbourg, France. European Pharmacopoeia Online 10.4; 2020.

[4] S. Görög, The importance and the challenges of impurity profiling in modern pharmaceutical analysis. TrAC. 2006, 25, 755-757.

[5] S. Görög, Critical review of reports on impurity and degradation product profiling in the last decade. TrAC. 2018, 101, 2-16.

[6] F. Sörgel, M. Kinzig, M. Abdel-Tawab, C. Bidmon, A. Schreiber, S. Ermel, J. Wohlfart, A. Besa, O. Scherf-Clavel, U. Holzgrabe, The contamination of valsartan and other sartans, part 1: New findings. J. Pharm. Biomed. Anal. 2019, 172, 395-405.

[7] M. Abdel-Tawab, R. Gröner, T. Kopp, J. Meins, J. Wübert, ZL findet NDMA in Tabletten. PZ Pharm. Ztg. 2018, 30, Available from: https://www.pharmazeutische-zeitung. de/index.php?id=77660. Accessed: September 28th 2020.

[8] EDQM, Strasbourg, France. Monograph No. 2423 - Valsartan. European Pharmacopoeia Online 10.4, 2020.

[9] T.K. Kishimoto, K. Viswanathan, T. Ganguly, S. Elankumaran, S. Smith, K. Pelzer, J.C. Lansing, N. Sriranganathan, G. Zhao, Z. Galcheva-Gargova, A. Al-Hakim, G.S. Bailey, B. Fraser, S. Roy, T. Rogers-Cotrone, L. Buhse, M. Whary, J. Fox, M. Nasr, G.J. Dal Pan, Z. Shriver, R.S. Langer, G. Venkataraman, K.F. Austen, J. Woodcock, R. Sasisekharan, Contaminated Heparin Associated

with Adverse Clinical Events and Activation of the Contact System. N. Engl. J. Med. 2008, 358, 2457-2467.

[10] S. Beni, J.F.K. Limtiaco, C.K. Larive, Analysis and characterization of heparin impurities. Anal. Bioanal. Chem. 2011, 399, 527-539.

[11] B. Mulloy, J. Hogwood, E. Gray, R. Lever, C.P. Page, Pharmacology of Heparin and Related Drugs. Pharmacol. Rev. 2016, 68, 76-141.

[12] R. Holm, D.P. Elder, Analytical advances in pharmaceutical impurity profiling. Eur. J. Pharm. Sci. 2016, 87, 118-135.

[13] EDQM, Strasbourg, France. Chapter 2.2.46 – Chromatographic Separation Techniques. European Pharmacopoeia Online 10.4, 2020.

[14] EDQM, Strasbourg, France. Chapter 2.2.29 – Liquid Chromatography. European Pharmacopoeia Online 10.4, 2020.

[15] L.R. Snyder, J.J. Kirkland, J.W. Dolan, Introduction to Modern Liquid Chromatography, 3rd ed., Wiley, Hoboken, New Jersey, 2010.

[16] D.A. Skoog, F.J. Holler, S.R. Crouch, Instrumentelle Analytik, 6. Auflage, Springer Spektrum, Berlin/Heidelberg, 2013.

[17] L.-E. Magnusson, D.S. Risley, J.A. Koropchak, Aerosol-based detectors for liquid chromatography. J. Chromatogr. A 2015, 1421, 68-81.

[18] B. Davani, Common Methods in Pharmaceutical Analysis. Pharmaceutical Analysis for Small Molecules, Wiley, Hoboken, 2017.

[19] M.W. Dong, D. Guillarme, Newer developments in HPLC impacting pharmaceutical analysis: A brief review. Am. Pharm. Rev. 2013, 16, 36-43.

[20] M.R. Siddiqui, Z.A. AlOthman, N. Rahman, Analytical techniques in pharmaceutical analysis: A review. Arab. J. Chem. 2017, 10, 1409-1421.

[21] EDQM, Strasbourg, France. Chapter 2.2.47 – Capillary Electrophoresis. European Pharmacopoeia Online 10.4, 2020.

[22] H.-F. Fan, F. Li, R.N. Zare, K-C. Lin, Characterization of two types of silanol groups on fused-silica surfaces using evanescent-wave cavity ring-down spectroscopy. Anal. Chem. 2007, 79, 3654-3661.

[23] X. Liu, J. Cheng, X. Lu, R. Wang, Surface acidity of quartz: understanding the crystallographic control. Phys. Chem. Chem. Phys. 2014, 16, 26909-26916.

[24] P.M. Nowak, M. Woźniakiewicz, M. Gładysz, M. Janus, P. Kościelniak, Improving repeatability of capillary electrophoresis – a critical comparison of ten different capillary inner surfaces and three criteria of peak identification. Anal. Bioanal. Chem. 2017, 409, 4383-4393.

[25] L. Hajba, A. Guttman, Recent advances in column coatings for capillary electrophoresis of proteins. TrAC. 2017, 90, 38-44.

[26] H. Engelhardt, W. Beck, T. Schmitt, Kapillarelektrophorese, Vieweg Verlag, Braunschweig/Wiesbaden, 1994.

[27] J. Wahl, U. Holzgrabe, Ionic liquids in capillary electrophoresis. Methods Mol. Biol. 2016, 1483, 131-153.

[28] L.G. Blomberg, H. Wan, Determination of enantiomeric excess by capillary electrophoresis. Electrophoresis 2000, 21, 1940-1952.

[29] P.T.T. Ha, J. Hoogmartens, A. Van Schepdael, Recent advances in pharmaceutical applications of chiral capillary electrophoresis. J. Pharm. Biomed. Anal. 2006, 41, 1-11.

[30] E. Sánchez-López, M.L. Marina, A.L. Crego, Improving the sensitivity in chiral capillary electrophoresis. Electrophoresis 2016, 37, 19-34.

[31] D. Moreno-Gonzáles, I. Lupión-Enríquez, A.M. García-Campaña, Trace determination of tetracyclines in water samples by capillary zone electrophoresis combining off-line and on-line preconcentration. Electrophoresis 2016, 37, 1212-1219.

[32] L. Suntornsuk, Recent advances of capillary electrophoresis in pharmaceutical analysis. Anal. Bioanal. Chem. 2010, 398, 29-52.

[33] R. Řemínek, F. Foret, Capillary electrophoretic methods for quality control analyses of pharmaceuticals: a review. Electrophoresis 2020, 0, 1-19.

[34] Z. Juvancz, R.B. Kendrovics, R. Iványi, L. Szente, The role of cyclodextrins in chiral capillary electrophoresis. Electrophoresis 2008, 29, 1701-1712.

[35] J. Kraly, M.A. Fazal, R.M. Schoenherr, R. Bonn, M.M. Harwood, E. Turner, M. Jones, N.J. Dovichi, Bioanalytical Applications of Capillary Electrophoresis. Anal. Chem. 2006, 78, 4097-4110.

[36] A.E. Derome, Modern NMR Techniques for Chemistry Research. Pergamon Press, Oxford, 1987.

[37] R.M. Maggio, N.L. Calvo, S.E. Vignaduzzo, T.S. Kaufman, Pharmaceutical impurities and degradation products: Uses and applications of NMR techniques. J. Pharm. Biomed. Anal. 2014, 101, 102-122.

[38] F. Malz, H. Jancke, Validation of quantitative NMR. J. Pharm. Biomed. Anal. 2005, 38, 813-823.

[39] B. King, The practical realization of the traceability of chemical measurements standards. Accred. Qual. Assur. 2000, 5, 429-436.

[40] B. King, Metrology in chemistry: Part II. Future requirements in Europe. Accred. Qual. Assur. 2000, 5, 266-271.

[41] U. Holzgrabe, Quantitative NMR spectroscopy in pharmaceutical applications. Progr. Nucl. Magn. Reson. Spectrosc. 2010, 57, 229-240.

[42] P. Giraudeau, I. Tea, G.S. Reamaud, S. Akoka, Reference and normalization methods: Essential tools for the intercomparison of NMR spectra. J. Pharm. Biomed. Anal. 2014, 93, 3-16.

[43] EDQM, Strasbourg, France. Chapter 2.2.33 - Nuclear Magnetic Resonance Spectrometry. European Pharmacopoeia Online 10.4, 2020.

[44] S.K. Bharti, R. Roy, Quantitative [1]H NMR spectroscopy. TrAC. 2012, 35, 5-26.

[45] G. Wider, L. Dreier, Measuring Protein Concentrations by NMR Spectroscopy. J. Am. Chem. Soc. 2006, 128, 2571-2576.

[46] Y.B. Monakhova, M. Kohl-Himmelseher, T. Kuballa, D.W. Lachenmeier, Determination of the purity of pharmaceutical reference materials by [1]H NMR using the standardless PULCON methodology. J. Pharm. Biomed. Anal. 2014, 100, 381-386.

[47] M. Hohmann, C. Felbinger, N. Christoph, H. Wachter, J. Wiest, U. Holzgrabe, Quantification of taurine in energy drinks using [1]H NMR. J. Pharm. Biomed. Anal. 2014, 93, 156-160.

[48] H.P. Mahon, Calibration system for a pulse nuclear induction spectrometer. Rev. Sci. Instrum. 1969, 40, 1644-1645.

[49] N. Zoelch, A. Hock, S. Heinzer-Schweizer, N. Avdievitch, A. Henning, Accurate determination of brain metabolite concentrations using ERETIC as external reference. NMR Biomed. 2017, 30, 3731.

[50] G.K. Pierens, A.R. Carroll, R.A. Davis, M.E. Palframan, R.J. Quinn, Determination of Analyte Concentration Using the Residual Solvent Resonance in [1]H NMR Spectroscopy. J. Nat. Prod. 2008, 71, 810-813.

[51] H. Mo, K.M. Balko, D.A. Colby, A practical deuterium-free NMR method for the rapid determination of 1-octanol/water partition coefficients of pharmaceutical agents. Bioorg. Med. Chem. Lett. 2010, 20, 6712-6715.

[52] B. Diehl, U. Holzgrabe, Analysis of drugs, in: U. Holzgrabe, B. Diehl, I. Wawer (Eds.), NMR Spectroscopy in Drug Development and Analysis, Wiley-VCH, Weinheim, 1999.

[53] U. Holzgrabe, R. Deubner, C. Schollmayer, B. Waibel, Quantitative NMR spectroscopy – Applications in drug analysis. J. Pharm. Biomed. Anal. 2005, 38, 806-812.

[54] U. Holzgrabe, I. Wawer, B. Diehl (Eds.), NMR Spectroscopy in Pharmaceutical Analysis, 1st ed., Elsevier, Oxford, UK, 2008.

[55] EDQM, Strasbourg, France. Chapter 2.2.64 – Peptide Identification By Nuclear Magnetic Resonance Spectrometry. European Pharmacopoeia Online 10.4, 2020.

[56] EDQM, Strasbourg, France. Monograph No. 0332 – Heparin calcium. European Pharmacopoeia Online 10.4, 2020.

[57] EDQM, Strasbourg, France. Monograph No. 0333 – Heparin sodium. European Pharmacopoeia Online 10.4, 2020.

[58] EDQM, Strasbourg, France. Monograph No. 0828 – Heparins, Low-Molecular-Mass. European Pharmacopoeia Online 10.4, 2020.

[59] EDQM, Strasbourg, France. Monograph No. 2046 – Lauromacrogol 400. European Pharmacopoeia Online 10.4, 2020.

[60] D. Parker, NMR Determination of Enantiomeric Purity. Chem. Rev. 1991, 91, 1441-1457.

[61] A.F. Casy, Chiral discrimination by NMR spectroscopy. TrAC. 1993, 12, 185-189.

[62] T.J. Wenzel, J.D. Wilcox, Chiral Reagents for the Determination of Enantiomeric Excess and Absolute Configuration Using NMR Spectroscopy. Chirality 2003, 15, 256-270.

[63] A. Cavazzini, L. Pasti, A. Massi, N. Marchetti, F. Dondi, Recent applications in chiral high performance liquid chromatography: A review. Anal. Chim. Acta 2011, 706, 205-222.

[64] V. Schurig, Separation of enantiomers by gas chromatography. J. Chromatogr. A 2001, 906, 275-299.

[65] B. Chankvetadze, W. Lindner, G.K.E. Scriba, Enantiomer Separations in Capillary Electrophoresis in the Case of Equal Binding Constants of the Enantiomers with a Chiral Selector: Commentary on the Feasibility of the Concept. Anal. Chem. 2004, 76, 4256-4260.

[66] R.B. Yu, J.P. Quirino, Chiral Selectors in Capillary Electrophoresis: Trends during 2017-2018. Molecules 2019, 24, 1135.

[67] G. Gübitz, M.G. Schmid, Chiral separation principles in capillary electrophoresis. J. Chromatogr. A 1997, 792, 179-225.

[68] Y. Liu, L.L. Sombra, P.W. Stege, Enantiomeric separation of β-blockers and tryptophan using heparin as stationary and pseudostationary phases in capillary electrophoresis. Chirality 2018, 30, 988-995.

[69] D.G.I. Kingston, Modern Natural Products Drug Discovery and Its Relevance to Biodiversity Conservation. J. Nat. Prod. 2011, 74, 496-511.

[70] J.W.-H. Li, J.C. Vederas, Drug Discovery and Natural Products: End of an Era or an Endless Frontier? Science 2009, 325, 161-165.

[71] Kommentar zum Europäischen Arzneibuch, Monographie 6.1/0097 – Morphinhydrochlorid. 52. Aktualisierungslieferung, Wissenschaftliche Verlagsgesellschaft Stuttgart, Stuttgart, 2015.

[72] Hochraffinierte Mineralöle in Kosmetika: Gesundheitliche Risiken sind nach derzeitigem Kenntnisstand nicht zu erwarten. Aktualisierte Stellungnahme Nr. 008/2018 des BfR, 27. Februar 2018.

[73] EDQM, Strasbourg, France. Monograph No. 1799 – Paraffin, White Soft. European Pharmacopoeia Online 10.4, 2020.

[74] EDQM, Strasbourg, France. Monograph No. 1554 – Paraffin, Yellow Soft. European Pharmacopoeia Online 10.4, 2020.

[75] EDQM, Strasbourg, France. Monograph No. 0239 – Paraffin, Liquid. European Pharmacopoeia Online 10.4, 2020.

[76] EDQM, Strasbourg, France. Monograph No. 0240 – Paraffin, Light Liquid. European Pharmacopoeia Online 10.4, 2020.

[77] EDQM, Strasbourg, France. Monograph No. 1034 – Paraffin, Hard. European Pharmacopoeia Online 10.4, 2020.

[78] International Council for Harmonization, Guideline Q3A(R2): Impurities in New Drug Substances 2006.

[79] S.L. Prabu, T.N.K. Suriyaprakash, Impurities and its importance in pharmacy. Int. J. Pharm. Sci. Rev. Res. 2010, 3, 66-71.

[80] International Council for Harmonization, Guideline Q1A(R2): Stability Testing Of New Drug Substances and Products 2003.

[81] International Council for Harmonization, Guideline Q1B: Stability Testing: Photostability Testing of New Drug Substances and Products 1996.

[82] International Council for Harmonization, Guideline Q5C: Quality of Biotechnological Products: Stability Testing of Biotechnological/Biological Products 1995.

[83] D. Jain, P.K. Basniwal, Forced degradation and impurity profiling: Recent trends in analytical perspectives. J. Pharm. Biomed. Anal. 2013, 86, 11-35.

[84] S.R. Bryn, W. Xu, A.W. Newman, Chemical reactivity in solid-state pharmaceuticals: formulation implications. Adv. Drug Del. Rev. 2001, 48, 115-136.

[85] M. Blessy, R.D. Patel, P.N. Prajapati, Y.K. Agrawal, Development of forced degradation and stability indicating studies of drugs – a review. J. Pharm. Anal. 2014, 4, 159-165.

[86] W. Kessler, Multivariate Datenanalyse, 1. Auflage, Wiley-VCH, Weinheim, 2007.

[87] EDQM, Strasbourg, France. Chapter 5.21 – Chemometric Methods Applied To Analytical Data. European Pharmacopoeia Online 10.4, 2020.

[88] A. Biancolillo, F. Marini, Chemometric Methods for Spectroscopy-Based Pharmaceutical Analysis. Front. Chem. 2018, 6, 1-14.

[89] Y.B. Monakhova, U. Holzgrabe, B.W.K. Diehl, Current role and future perspectives of multivariate (chemometric) methods in NMR spectroscopic analysis of pharmaceutical products. J. Pharm. Biomed. Anal. 2018, 147, 580-589.

[90] S. Matero, F. van Den Berg, S. Poutiainen, J. Rantanen, J. Pajander, Towards better process understanding: chemometrics and multivariate measurements in manufacturing of solide dosage forms. J. Pharm. Sci. 2013, 102, 1385-1403.

[91] S. Challa, R. Potumarthi, Chemometrics-based process analytical technology (PAT) tools: applications and adaption in pharmaceutical and biopharmaceutical industries. Appl. Biochem. Biotechnol. 2013, 169, 66-76.

# 2. Aim of the book

For the quality control of APIs and excipients, a variety of different methods for pharmaceutical analysis were applied in this doctoral book.

Drugs and excipients deriving from natural sources are often multi-component mixtures. Purity evaluation can be very challenging, since a particular compound or a group of compounds has to be determined and quantified in a suitable way. Paraffins as mineral oil derived mixtures of hydrocarbon molecules should be analyzed to evaluate the amount of the residual mineral oil aromatic hydrocarbons, which may be potentially carcinogenic. Therefore, a suitable $^1$H NMR method was developed and applied on various paraffin samples. The results should be compared to a former compendial UV method and evaluated by means of principal component analysis.

The impurity profile of L-ascorbic acid 2-phosphate magnesium (A2PMg) was characterized by derivatives with different phosphate substitutions. This was examined by means of one- and multidimensional $^1$H, $^{13}$C and $^{31}$P NMR spectroscopy.

Stability testing of APIs is necessary to monitor their quality under varying environmental factors as described by the ICH guideline Q1A(R2). Degradation products may be formed by decomposition or isomerization of the former drug and need to be investigated. Stress tests may accelerate the formation of the degradation products and can be conducted under basic, acidic, oxidizing and/or light intense conditions in solid state or in solution. The aim was to examine the degradation of APIs which were stressed in a ball mill under solid state conditions. As one part, the isomerization of dexibuprofen was evaluated. Therefore, an enantioselective capillary electrophoresis method was developed, validated and applied on stressed samples. In the other part, the degradation profile of oxidatively stressed clopidogrel was examined by means of HPLC-UV and HPLC-MS(/MS).

# 3. Results

## 3.1 Characterization of mineral oil hydrocarbons in paraffins for pharmaceutical use by means of [1]H NMR and UV spectroscopy and principal component analysis

### 3.1.1 [1]H NMR analytical characterization of Mineral Oil Hydrocarbons (PARAFFINS) for Pharmaceutical Use

Jonas Urlaub, Jochen Norwig, Curd Schollmayer, Ulrike Holzgrabe



**Abstract**

Mineral oil hydrocarbons incorporated in pharmaceutical preparations are frequently administered to the skin as creams and/or ointments. However, the oral route is also of interest when the substances are used in form of medicated lip sticks or for the polishing of coated tablets. In Europe, the substances are monographed by the European Pharmacopoeia as Liquid Paraffin, Light Liquid Paraffin, White Soft Paraffin, Yellow Soft Paraffin, and Hard Paraffin. The consistency differs from liquid and semi-solid to solid and influences the functional characteristics. Because these excipients are produced from petroleum, they contain residual traces of aromatic compounds. Therefore, the European Pharmacopoeia tests the substances on residual impurities of condensed poly aromatic hydrocarbons. Recently, the question arose whether these tests are fully sufficient, since toxic condensed polyaromatic hydrocarbons are only one type of aromatic compounds found in mineral oil hydrocarbons. Especially aliphatic hydrocarbons containing isolated spots of aromatic cores are not in the focus of compendial tests. Therefore, combined chromatographic methods were developed and should resolve this problem by a separation of the different aromatic impurities. Because these chromatographic techniques involve several steps and the interpretation of the result is difficult, we established a quantitative $^1$H NMR spectroscopic method for the determination of aromatic traces in mineral oil hydrocarbons. The technique is a holistic approach for all traces of aromatic hydrocarbons. The technique was tested with several samples collected from different stages of the refinement process and in addition with different excipient samples from the market. Moreover, a few samples of synthetic paraffin made by the Fischer-Tropsch process were analyzed. The results reveal the purification characteristics of the refinement and the differences in the aromatic impurities.

## 1. Introduction

Mineral oil hydrocarbons (MOH) are a group of substances consisting of mixtures of heterogeneous hydrocarbon molecules which may include saturated and/or unsaturated hydrocarbons with a linear, branched, or cyclic structure. The number of carbon atoms is varying in a wide range. The main basic structures are n-, iso-, and cycloalkanes as well as aromatic compounds. Naturally occurring hydrocarbons are primarily n-alkanes of an odd-number of carbon atoms from $C_{21}$ to $C_{35}$, including terpenoids and oligomeric hydrocarbons released from polyolefins, largely consisting of branched alkanes (Fig. 1).

Paraffins and naphthenes – cycloalkanes – are abbreviated as MOSH (mineral oil saturated hydrocarbons), whereas aromatic hydrocarbons are called MOAH (mineral oil aromatic hydrocarbons – Fig. 1). Additionally, the paraffins/naphthenes intended for pharmaceutical use are classified according to their carbon chain length and viscosity, measured at 100 °C [1]: medium & low viscosity ($C_{10}$ - $C_{25}$), high viscosity (> $C_{30}$), microcrystalline waxes, and solid paraffins ($C_{20}$ - $C_{60}$). Petroleum (crude mineral oil) is by far considered as the predominant source of the MOH, but physicochemically equivalent products can also be synthesized from coal, natural gas, or biomass. The composition of the products is predetermined either by the petroleum which is used as starting material or by the treatment during refining such as distillation, extraction, cracking, or hydro-treatment [2]. Moreover, the addition of hydrocarbons from other or different sources is intended in order to get the desired functional related characteristics (FRC). The composition of functionally equivalent products may differ substantially, depending on the way they were obtained.

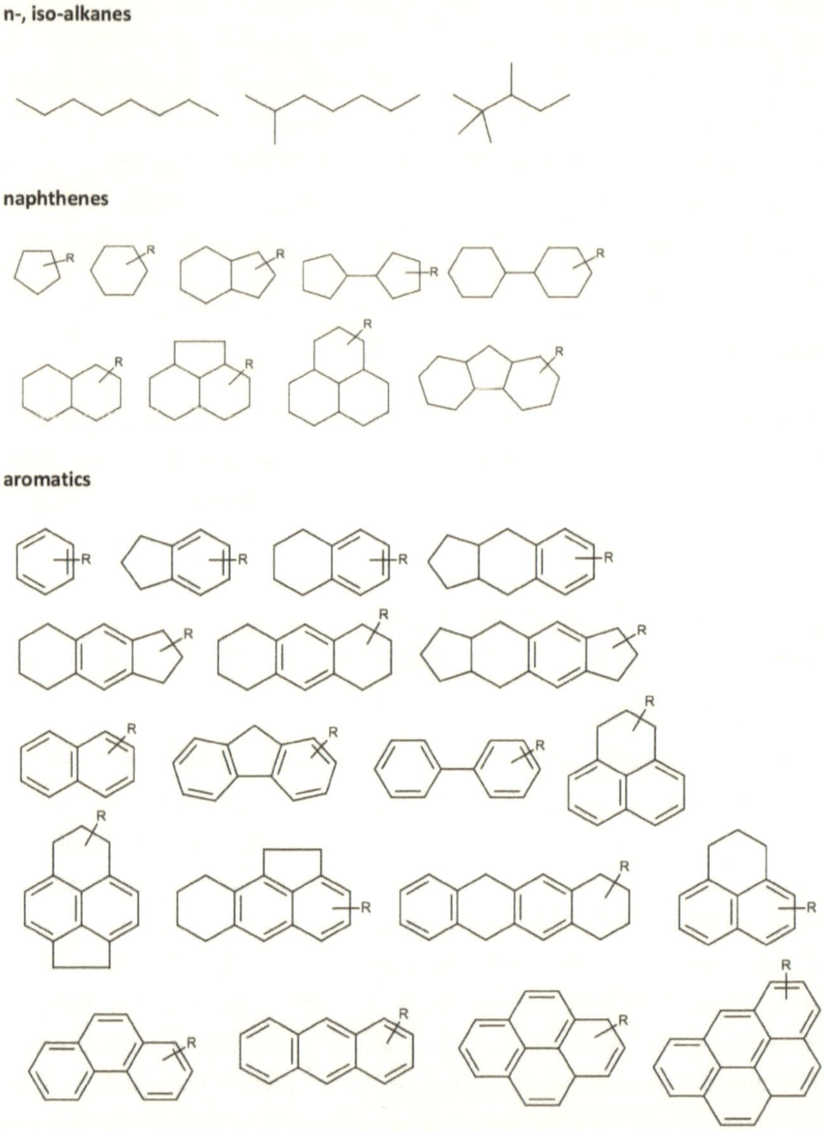

<sup>1</sup>H NMR analytical characterization of Mineral Oil Hydrocarbons (PARAFFINS) for Pharmaceutical Use

**n-, iso-alkanes**

**naphthenes**

**aromatics**

**Fig. 1.** Different structural moieties of MOH. R = alkanes, alkenes C10 - C100+.

## 1.1 Petroleum processing – refining and purification process

As mentioned before, the origin of the petroleum predetermines the viscosity and composition of the raw material. Consequently, the refineries need to adapt the refinery process accordingly. Nevertheless, several principal processes do not differ on the pathway from the feedstock to the intermediate raw material of the MOH production for pharmaceutical use. Most important for producing the pharmaceutical grade MOH (Paraffins) is the processing of the heavy distillates and residues of the atmospheric distillation. The residue is further treated by a vacuum distillation and several refinements such as solvent extraction, solvent dewaxing, hydrocracking, and dearomatization. Referring to the viscosity and physical state of the PARAFFIN of pharmaceutical grade, a different refining of the liquid fraction or the solid fraction of this vacuum distillation is performed. From the liquid fractions, light liquid paraffin and liquid paraffin (European Pharmacopoeia – Ph.Eur. [3,4]) are gained. From the solid wax fraction, hard paraffin (Ph.Eur. [5]) and microcrystalline wax (formerly in USP [6]) are obtained. The semi-solid substances white soft paraffin (Ph.Eur. [7]) and yellow soft paraffin (Ph.Eur. [8]) are carefully designed blends of solid and liquid fractions according to the desired functional properties [9]. Removing and diminishing of undesired compounds is a major prerequisite for the pharmaceutical use. The refining details, the composition and the manufacturing of all pharmaceutical relevant paraffin excipients are described in [10].

The process of solvent extraction physically separates the aromatic hydrocarbons and minor compounds of higher polarity. The product obtained contains almost all saturated hydrocarbons from the initial distillate, about 1/3 of the aromatic and polar molecules, and only a few percent of the initial polycyclic aromatic hydrocarbons (PAH).

The dewaxing physically removes the linear alkanes or waxes to obtain a free flowing and homogeneous liquid at 0 °C. The impact on composition is an almost complete removal of linear waxes, a reduction of little-branched isoparaffins, balanced by a slight, proportional increase of other hydrocarbon types and polar residues.

Optional hydrocracking removes waxes by selective cracking of linear molecules over a chemical shape-selective catalyst at high temperature (300 to 360 °C) and under medium to high hydrogen pressure.

Dearomatization treats the feedstock as obtained from the previous steps with an excess of sulfur trioxide or fuming sulfuric acid (oleum) in a stirred reactor. The aromatic hydrocarbons react with the sulfur trioxide or oleum to yield arylsulfonic acids; the S-, N- and O-containing molecules are decomposed, oxidized, or neutralized. Although most of the aromatic hydrocarbons and impurities are removed, the process is not quantitative and the oily phase is then returned for additional oleum (concentrated sulfuric acid) treatment. The process is continued until all molecules being reactive with sulfuric acid are removed.

## 1.2 Pharmaceutical use of purified paraffins

Only refined and purified paraffins are used as pharmaceutical excipients for cutaneous use. Similar to the cutaneous use, the administration of pharmaceutical grade paraffin to several mucous membranes in dosage forms for gingival, rectal, or vaginal use is applied. Lip sticks also contain purified paraffins like hard paraffin. Table 1 represents an overview of the routes of administration seen on the German market.

A query on the data base (Arzneimittel Informationssystem – AMIS) of the German health authorities is the source for the tabulated values and the additional information in Table 1. Referring to the toxicological evaluation of the substances, the oral ingestion is most critical and should be reduced as much as possible.

## 1.3 Quality assessment of paraffins

For the toxicological testing and the quality analytical purposes, the PAH and PAC fraction could be extracted from paraffin intermediates by dimethyl sulfoxide. DMSO (dimethyl sulfoxide) is an appropriate solvent with a high affinity to these compounds [12]. This is the background for the pharmacopoeial UV tests on PAH or PAC which were introduced at the beginning of the 90[th]s. Whereas the PAC are limited by the pharmacopoeial test methods, MOAH are not tested by a specific pharmacopoeial test.

In pharmaceutical and cosmetic industries, the analysis of MOSH and MOAH is mostly performed using an on-line coupled high performance liquid chromatography-gas chromatography-flame ionization detection (HPLC-GC-FID). This application was comprehensively described by Biedermann et al. [13,14]. A different ¹H NMR approach for determining MOAH and MOSH in mineral oil-based products was reported by Lachenmeier et al. [15], using the PULCON (Pulse length-based concentration determination) methodology. From the analytical point of view, the application of simple 1D $^1$H NMR spectroscopy is a comprehensive and sufficient tool to control the desired refining of all aromatic MOH. The aromatic constituents of the products were analyzed by $^1$H NMR spectroscopy, and the ratio of the integrals of aromatic and aliphatic signals, representing MOAH and MOSH, were used to control the quality of mineral oil hydrocarbons.

**Table 1.** Number of pharmaceutical preparations containing purified PARAFFINs on the German market listed with the estimated MOAH contact per day.

| Substance | No. of pharmaceutical preparations | typical use | special use | estimated MOAH contact per day | background exposure per day by food [11] |
|---|---|---|---|---|---|
| Paraffinum perliquidum (Light Liquid Paraffin) | 159 | cutaneous | oral | 0.01 µg per oral dose | 420 - 4200 µg |
| Paraffinum liquidum (Liquid Paraffin) | 374 | cutaneous | oral | 0.0015 µg per oral dose | 420 - 4200 µg |
| Vaselinum Album (White Soft Paraffin) | 762 | cutaneous | not for oral use | ≤ 1000 µg per cutaneous dose | 420 - 4200 µg |
| Paraffinum durum (Hard Paraffin) | 79 | cutaneous | oral | ≤ 0.01 µg per oral dose | 420 - 4200 µg |

## 2. Materials and method

### 2.1 Samples, materials and test solutions

The manufacturers of the paraffin excipients use a different nomenclature and in addition, trade names give a terminological hint which type of paraffin is meant. In the following jelly, Vaseline and petrolatum are used in trade names as synonyms of White Soft Paraffin. The expression Vaseline belongs to White Soft Paraffin whereas Petrolatum is the term used by the USP. Jelly is a non-compendial term for White Soft Paraffin and is used solely by the manufacturers in their trade names.

The analyzed samples were provided by Sasol Wax, Shell Global Solutions, European Wax Federation, Tudapetrol KG, Aiglon, H&R (Hansen & Rosenthal) KG, Sonneborn, Alpha Wax, and local pharmacies. An overview of all samples is given in Table 2. Chloroform-d ($CDCl_3$, 99.96 atom % D, with and without TMS 0.03% V/V) and dichloromethane-$d_2$ ($CD_2Cl_2$, 99.9 atom % D, with and without TMS 0.1% V/V) were purchased from Sigma-Aldrich (Schnelldorf, Germany). All samples were measured in Norell 5 mm o.d., 507-HP-7 NMR tubes (Morganton, USA).

The test solutions for $^1$H NMR measurements were prepared as follows: 25 mg of the respective semi-solid sample was dissolved in a mixture of 900 µL of $CDCl_3$ and 100 µL of $CDCl_3$ containing tetramethylsilane (TMS, 0.03% V/V), and vortexed for about 1 minute. 700 µL of the solution were transferred into a 5 mm NMR tube for measurement. For the preparation of the solution of liquid paraffin samples, 100 mg of the analyte was dissolved in a mixture of 970 µL $CD_2Cl_2$ and 30 µL $CD_2Cl_2$ containing TMS (0.1% V/V). After thoroughly shaking the mixture, 700 µL were transferred into a 5 mm NMR tube. For the test solutions of the respective solid paraffin samples, 25 mg of the synthetic solid paraffin samples and 100 mg of the hard paraffin sample was dissolved in a mixture of 900 µL $CDCl_3$ and 100 µL $CDCl_3$ containing TMS (0.03% V/V). After homogenizing the solution, 700 µL were transferred into a 5 mm NMR tube for measurement.

**Table 2.** Paraffin samples to be tested.

| Sample No. | Sample ID | Labelling | Content | Manufacturer |
| --- | --- | --- | --- | --- |
| 1 | CJMS | Carisma Jelly MediumSoft | soft paraffin | Alpha Wax |
| 2 | CJSS | Carisma Jelly SilkySoft | soft paraffin | Alpha Wax |
| 3 | CJUS | Carisma Jelly UltraSoft | soft paraffin | Alpha Wax |
| 4 | FT1 | #HLA 3091 | soft paraffin | Sonneborn |
| 5 | FT2 | #HLA 3092 | soft paraffin | Sonneborn |
| 6 | FT3 | #HLA 3093 | soft paraffin | Sonneborn |
| 7 | A | Sample A | soft paraffin | European Wax Federation |
| 8 | B | Sample B | soft paraffin | European Wax Federation |
| 9 | C | Sample C | soft paraffin | European Wax Federation |
| 10 | D | Sample D | soft paraffin | European Wax Federation |
| 11 | E | Sample E | soft paraffin | European Wax Federation |
| 12 | F | Sample F | soft paraffin | European Wax Federation |
| 13 | G | Sample G | soft paraffin | European Wax Federation |
| 14 | H | Sample H | soft paraffin | European Wax Federation |
| 15 | K | Sample K | soft paraffin | European Wax Federation |
| 16 | L | Sample L | soft paraffin | European Wax Federation |
| 17 | M | Sample M | soft paraffin | European Wax Federation |
| 18 | A1 | Sample A1 | soft paraffin | Sasol Wax |
| 19 | A2 | Sample A2 | soft paraffin | Sasol Wax |
| 20 | B1 | Sample B1 | soft paraffin | Sasol Wax |

**Table 2.** (Continued)

| 21 | B2 | Sample B2 | soft paraffin | Sasol Wax |
|---|---|---|---|---|
| 22 | C1 | Sample C1 | soft paraffin | Sasol Wax |
| 23 | C2 | Sample C2 | soft paraffin | Sasol Wax |
| 24 | SW H1 | Sasolwax H1 | solid paraffin | Sasol Wax |
| 25 | SW 2699 | Sasolwax 2699 | solid paraffin | Sasol Wax |
| 26 | SW 2700 | Sasolwax 2700 | solid paraffin | Sasol Wax |
| 27 | SW 3279 | Sasolwax 3279 | solid paraffin | Sasol Wax |
| 28 | TV1 | Technical vaseline 1 | soft paraffin | Tudapetrol KG |
| 29 | TV2 | Technical vaseline 2 | soft paraffin | Tudapetrol KG |
| 30 | TV3 | Technical vaseline 3 | soft paraffin | Tudapetrol KG |
| 31 | VA1 | Vaseline Aiglon 001 | soft paraffin | Aiglon |
| 32 | VA2 | Vaseline Aiglon 002 | soft paraffin | Aiglon |
| 33 | VA3 | Vaseline Aiglon 003 | soft paraffin | Aiglon |
| 34 | VasAlb | Vaselinum Album | soft paraffin | Caelo |
| 35 | VasFlav | Vaselinum Flavum | soft paraffin | Caelo |
| 36 | SN600D | Destillates Heavy Paraffine | paraffin intermediate | Shell Global Solutions GmbH |
| 37 | SN600WR | SN600 Waxy raffinate | paraffin intermediate | Shell Global Solutions GmbH |
| 38 | VP50268 GTL | Pionier VP 50268-GTL | soft paraffin | H&R KG |
| 39 | VP60200 3/7 | Pionier VP 60200-3/7 | soft paraffin | H&R KG |
| 40 | VP60216 3 | Pionier VP 60216-3 | soft paraffin | H&R KG |
| 41 | ParDur | Paraffinum durum | solid paraffin | Caelo |

**Table 2.** (Continued)

| 42 | ParPerl1 | Paraffinum perliquidum 1 | liquid paraffin | Caelo |
| 43 | ParPerl2 | Paraffinum perliquidum 2 | liquid paraffin | Caelo |
| 44 | ParLiq1 | Paraffinum liquidum 1 | liquid paraffin | Caelo |
| 45 | Parliq2 | Paraffinum liquidum 2 | liquid paraffin | Caelo |
| 46 | P2071 | Pionier 2071 | liquid paraffin | H&R Wax Company GmbH |
| 47 | P2076 | Pionier 2076 | liquid paraffin | H&R Wax Company GmbH |
| 48 | P6501 | Pionier 6501 | liquid paraffin | H&R Wax Company GmbH |
| 49 | OX415 | Ondina X 415 | liquid paraffin | Shell Global Solutions GmbH |
| 50 | OX420 | Ondina X 420 | liquid paraffin | Shell Global Solutions GmbH |
| 51 | OX430 | Ondina X 430 | liquid paraffin | Shell Global Solutions GmbH |
| 52 | SN600BO | SN600 Baseoil | paraffin intermediate | Shell Global Solutions GmbH |
| 53 | SN600MWO | SN600 Medical White Oil | liquid paraffin | Shell Global Solutions GmbH |
| 54 | SN600TWO | SN600 Technical White Oil | liquid paraffin | Shell Global Solutions GmbH |

## 2.2 Solubility testing

200 mg of the respective semi-solid/synthetic solid sample was weighed into a preparation vial and 1000 µL $CDCl_3$ added. Subsequently the mixture was intensely shaken. If no clear solution was obtained within 1 minute at 313 K, $CDCl_3$ was added in order to decrease the concentration of the analyte in 5 mg/mL steps until a clear solution resulted. For the even less soluble samples (< 5 mg/mL), a dilution to 1 mg/mL per test was applied.

## 2.3 NMR method

All measurements were performed using a Bruker Avance III 400 MHz UltraShield spectrometer equipped with a 5-mm PABBI ATM 1H/D-BB Z-GRD probe, a Bruker automatic sample changer (B-ACS 60), a BSVT (Bruker Smart Variable Temperature System), and a BCU05 (Bruker Cooling Unit). The measurements were conducted at 313 K for the soft and solid paraffin samples and at 293 K for the liquid paraffins. The temperature was adjusted to be constant over the measurements by using a thermometer sample of Methanol-$d_4$ 99.8%. All NMR spectra were recorded in the baseopt mode using the Bruker standard zg pulse sequence with a pulse angle of 90°, 256 scans (NS), and 2 prior dummy scans (DS). The spectral width (SW) was 30 ppm and the size of the fid (TD) was 128k. The acquisition time was 5.45 seconds followed by a relaxation delay (D1) of 10 seconds for the soft and synthetic solid paraffin samples, and 6 seconds for the liquid and hard paraffin samples, respectively. The measurements were performed without rotation. The receiver gain (RG) was kept constant at 32 for the soft/synthetic solid paraffin samples and at 5.6 for the liquid/hard paraffin samples. The chemical shifts were referred to the TMS signal. All spectra were processed using TopSpin 3.5.7 by Bruker. Both phase correction (0. order) and integration were performed manually. The baseline correction was done using the following areas: $\delta = 14 - 12$ ppm (noise area for determination of the signal to noise ratio [S/N]), $\delta = 10 - 6$ ppm (MOAH region), $\delta = 5 - (-2)$ ppm (for soft and synthetic solid paraffin) or $\delta = 5 - (-4)$ ppm (for liquid and hard paraffin).

# 3. Results

## 3.1 Optimization of the $^1$H NMR measurement

### 3.1.1 Choice of solvent and signal-to-noise-ratio

It is an essential issue to choose an appropriate solvent that features good dissolving characteristics on the one hand and no signal overlapping in the MOAH/MOSH region on the other hand. Liquid paraffin samples were measured in $CD_2Cl_2$. The advantage of this solvent is the lack of residual solvent signals in the range of the aromatic protons of the MOAH and the aliphatic protons of the MOSH. Unfortunately, $CD_2Cl_2$ is neither suitable for soft nor for hard paraffin analysis because of its insufficient dissolving capability. This is the reason why the measurement of the hard paraffin sample was performed in $CDCl_3$ instead. An obvious problem is the residual solvent signal of $CHCl_3$ which needs to be excluded from integration. Other solvents tested either showed residual solvent signals inside the interesting areas as well (hexane-$d_6$, benzene-$d_6$, impurities of $CCl_4$), or their dissolving capability is too low ($CD_2Cl_2$, $D_2O$). The advantage of using $CDCl_3$ is its acceptable solving feature on the one hand. On the other hand, the residual solvent signal can very easily be excluded in contrast to $CCl_4$ where multiple signals of impurities have to be considered.

An alternative approach to fix the problem of poor solubility was increasing the temperature to 313 K. To yield an acceptable signal-to-noise ratio (S/N) with respect to a preferably high amount of dissolved samples, a concentration of 25 mg/mL was chosen for measurements. Additionally, it is possible to increase the number of scans to improve the S/N ratio, but this resulted in unacceptable long measuring times. Here, 256 scans were applied, resulting in about 70 minutes per sample. For determining the S/N ratio it is important to exclude the $^{13}$C satellites of $CHCl_3$ from integration because they pretend much higher values; this is not necessary when using $CD_2Cl_2$.

### 3.1.2 Relaxation delay

For quantitative NMR analysis, protons of a substance studied are supposed to fully relax. This is generally achieved by setting the interscan delay to five times the value of the $T_1$ relaxation time [16]. $T_1$ was determined using an inversion-recovery experiment. The longest $T_1$ relaxation time of a proton within the MOAH region is about 3 seconds for semi-solid and synthetic paraffin samples (measured in $CDCl_3$) and 2 seconds for the liquid and hard paraffin samples (measured in $CD_2Cl_2$ and $CDCl_3$, respectively). Since the interscan delay consists of the acquisition time and the D1 time, fully relaxation was accomplished by setting the D1 value to 10 and 6 seconds, respectively. The acquisition time was 5.45 seconds.

### 3.1.3 Repeatability

The repeatability [17] was evaluated for the measurements of both semi-solid and liquid paraffin samples. 6 samples of "VP60200-3/7" (313 K, 25 mg/mL in $CDCl_3$) and "P2071" (293 K, 100 mg/mL in $CD_2Cl_2$) were measured, respectively. The relative standard deviation was about 0.82% for the semi-solid sample and 4.6% for the liquid paraffin sample, which is considered to be precise. The increased relative standard deviation of the liquid paraffin measurements is due to the low signal-to-noise ratios of the MOAH region. The receiver gain used for the liquid paraffin samples (5.6) was low compared to the semi-solid samples (32). This leads to a more complicated baseline correction of the spectrum. Both factors highly affect the integration process which is considered to be the main source of uncertainties.

### 3.2 Interpretation of $^1$H NMR spectra

A representative $^1$H NMR spectrum of soft paraffin is shown in Fig. 2. Basically, it is composed of two signal regions, the aromatic and the aliphatic one. Whereas the protons of a single phenyl ring typically resonate at $\delta = 7.26$ ppm with a slight upfield shift when carrying an alkyl chain ($\Delta\delta = 0.1$ to 0.2 ppm), polycyclic aromatic hydrogens are substantially downfield shifted: unsubstituted naphthalene gave signals at $\delta = 7.3$ and 7.6 ppm, anthracene at $\delta = 7.4$, 7.9, and 8.4 ppm, and phenanthrene between $\delta = 7.7$ to 8.9 ppm which can be further upfield shifted by alkylation [18]. Thus, the NMR spectra can provide information of the degree of condensation of the aromatic moieties of MOAH.

<sup></sup>¹H NMR analytical characterization of Mineral Oil Hydrocarbons (PARAFFINS) for Pharmaceutical Use

---

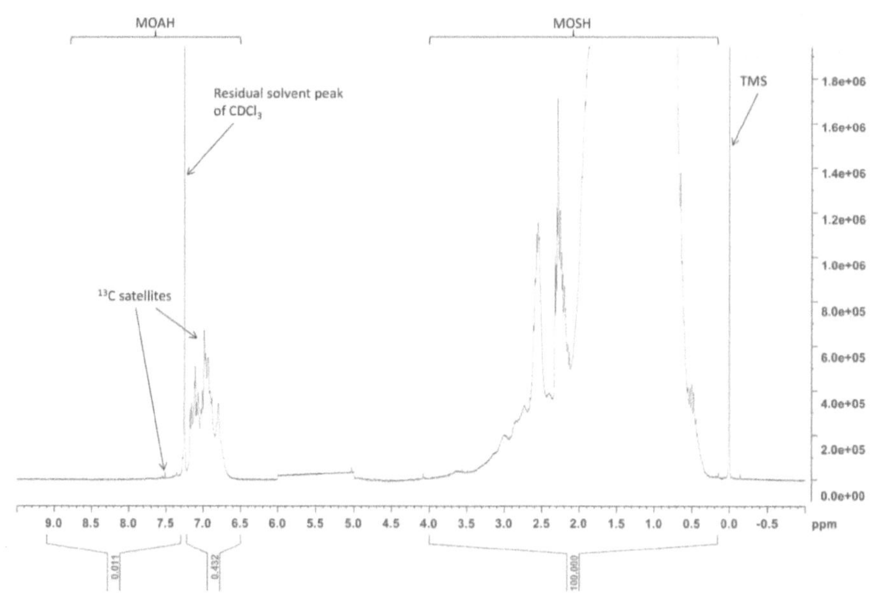



**Fig. 2.** Processed ¹H NMR spectrum of the semi-solid paraffin sample "sample D".

The integration of the aromatic part of the MOAH in the downfield region was performed between δ = 9.10 - 7.30 ppm and δ = 7.22 - 6.50 ppm, excluding the residual solvent peak of $CHCl_3$ at δ = 7.25 ppm. The aliphatic signals of the MOSH in the upfield region were integrated from δ = 4.00 - 0.16 ppm. There are two groups of signals that are located on the left shoulder of the MOSH region, representing the protons attached next to the aromatic structures (benzylic, methylene, and methyl groups). The signals between the aromatic and aliphatic regions represent other groups being neither MOSH nor MOAH. They belong to e.g. acrylates and unsaturated residues.

The term "aromatic/aliphatic ratio" (abbreviated as a/a ratios) which is used to describe the paraffin samples represents the ratio of the integrals of aromatic protons (MOAH) and the aliphatic protons (MOSH). Since the vast majority of protons belong to the aliphatic moieties (MOSH), no great errors are expected using this term.

¹H NMR spectra of a semi-solid paraffin sample measured in $CDCl_3$ and a liquid paraffin sample measured in $CD_2Cl_2$ are representatively depicted in Figs. 2 and 3. The residual solvent peak of $CD_2Cl_2$ at about δ = 5.36 ppm enables a gapless

integration of the MOAH from δ = 9.1 - 6.5 ppm. The MOSH region was integrated from δ = 4 - 0.16 ppm.

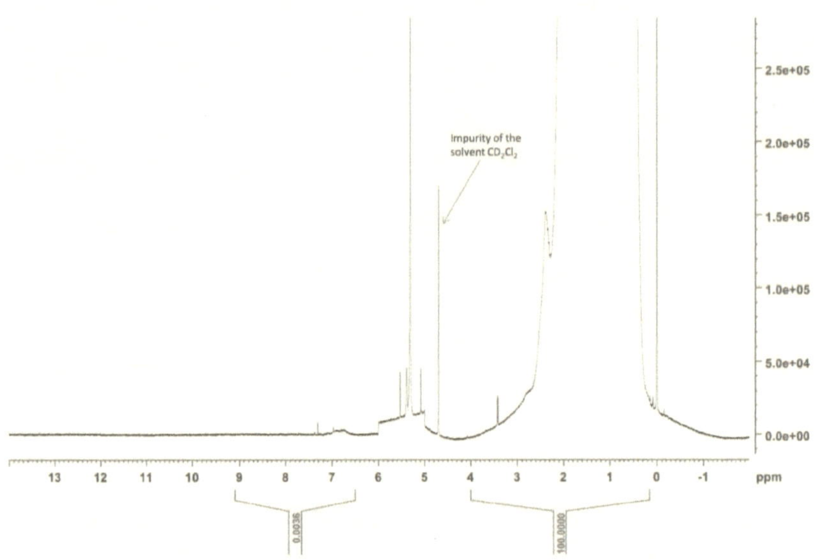


**Fig. 3.** Processed ¹H NMR spectrum of the liquid paraffin sample "Pionier 2071".

## 4. Discussion

A wide range of paraffin samples from different manufacturers was covered. Some products are not of pharmaceutical grade; they are intermediates of the production process or technical products. Hence, the sample pool is considered to have a high degree of diversity and is sensitive to reveal differences in the degree of aromatic impurities.

### 4.1 Semi-solid and solid synthetic paraffin measurements

The resulting aromatic-aliphatic ratios are displayed in Table 3 and represent the percentage of the aromatic protons in relation to the aliphatic protons. The a/a ratio of most of the samples is ranging between 0.02 and 0.5%. The sample "SN600D" has by far the highest MOAH content (3.77%). This dark, tar smelling distillate is an early intermediate in the manufacturing of mineral oil products and is directly obtained from vacuum distillation. The sample "SN600WR", in contrast, is a waxy raffinate that experienced an extraction step reducing the number of aromatic components. This sample is an intermediate product like "SN600D" and thus its MOAH content is still high (0.696%). The samples "A1", "B1", and "C1" show a/a values comparable to the "waxy raffinate" (Table 3). They have not been hydrogenated yet for removal of remaining MOAH. As expected, their hydrogenated counterparts (samples "A2", "B2", and "C2") show smaller a/a ratios of MOAH due to the hydrogenation process. As already described, the purification process of mineral oil products is often connected with its use. Technical soft paraffins for example (samples "TV1", "TV2", "TV3") show relative high amounts of MOAH compared to other measured soft paraffins (Table 3). However, compared to other samples like "D", "H", or "K", the MOAH contents of the technical soft paraffins are not substantially higher.

**Table 3.** Aromatic/aliphatic proton ratios of the respective samples, arranged in order of increasing a/a values.

| Description | Sample-ID | aromatic/aliphatic protons [%] | Solubility (313 K, CDCl$_3$) [mg/mL] |
| --- | --- | --- | --- |
| Synthetic Wax | SWH1 | 0 | <1 |
| Synthetic Wax | SW2699 | 0 | <1 |
| Microcrystalline Wax | SW3279 | 0.018 | <1 |
| White Soft Paraffin | C | 0.023 | 120 |
| White Soft Paraffin | VA1 | 0.025 | 20 |
| White Soft Paraffin | L | 0.027 | 65 |
| White Soft Paraffin | M | 0.027 | 65 |
| Synthetic Wax | SW2700 | 0.027 | <1 |
| White Soft Paraffin | VA2 | 0.044 | 20 |
| White Soft Paraffin | VA3 | 0.045 | 20 |
| White Soft Paraffin | CJMS | 0.053 | 200 |
| White Soft Paraffin | CJSS | 0.054 | 150 |
| White Soft Paraffin | VP60200-3/7 | 0.055 | 2.5 |
| White Soft Paraffin | VP60216-3 | 0.057 | 5 |
| White Soft Paraffin | CJUS | 0.067 | 200 |
| White Soft Paraffin | A | 0.075 | 45 |
| White Soft Paraffin | B | 0.077 | 160 |
| White Soft Paraffin | FT3 | 0.097 | 45 |

**Table 3.** (Continued)

| | | | |
|---|---|---|---|
| White Soft Paraffin | FT2 | 0.098 | 35 |
| White Soft Paraffin | FT1 | 0.099 | 50 |
| White Soft Paraffin | VP50268-GTL | 0.103 | 65 |
| White Soft Paraffin | E | 0.112 | 25 |
| White Soft Paraffin | G | 0.177 | 110 |
| Technical Soft Paraffin | TV3 | 0.180 | 25 |
| White Soft Paraffin | A2 | 0.193 | 35 |
| White Soft Paraffin | F | 0.215 | 40 |
| White Soft Paraffin | VasAlb | 0.216 | 10 |
| Technical Soft Paraffin | TV2 | 0.223 | 30 |
| White Soft Paraffin | H | 0.233 | 25 |
| White Soft Paraffin | K | 0.317 | 35 |
| Technical Soft Paraffin | TV1 | 0.383 | 30 |
| White Soft Paraffin | D | 0.444 | 60 |
| Yellow Soft Paraffin | VasFlav | 0.477 | 50 |
| White Soft Paraffin | C2 | 0.490 | 60 |
| White Soft Paraffin | B2 | 0.548 | 20 |
| Soft Paraffin | C1 | 0.686 | 60 |
| Paraffin intermediate | SN600WR | 0.696 | >>200 |
| Soft Paraffin | B1 | 0.767 | 20 |
| Soft Paraffin | A1 | 0.989 | 50 |
| Paraffin intermediate | SN600D | 3.770 | >>200 |

The four samples "SWH1", "SW2699", "SW2700", and "SW3279" were produced artificially. "SW3279" and "SWH1" are small, solid pellets like "paraffinum durum", "SW2699" and "SW2700" are white, greasy powders. As displayed in Table 3, "SWH1" and "SW2699" show no detectable MOAH signals, while "SW2700" and "SW3279" are observed to contain small amounts of MOAH.

Since soft paraffin is a heterogeneous mixture of hydrocarbon molecules, the solubility is expected to differ among the various samples when preparing the test solutions. The solubility of the soft paraffins was found to be an issue for some batches (Table 3). For instance, the sample "VasAlb" is not completely soluble at the measuring conditions (25 mg/mL in $CDCl_3$, 313 K). In this case, a formation of two phases within the sample solution was observed which means the upper turbid layer separates from the lower clear one. The two phases were measured separately by means of [1]H NMR and showed equal a/a ratios for both layers.

Besides evaluating the MOAH content, the solubility of the soft paraffin samples was determined (Table 3) and was found to cover a huge range. The samples "VasAlb", "60216-3" and "60200-3/7" show low solubility ($\leq$ 10 mg/mL), whereas the samples "B", "C", "G", "CJMS", "CJSS", "CJUS", "SN600D", and "SN600WR" were pretty soluble (> 100 mg/mL). Regarding groups of samples like the technical soft paraffins ("TV") or the Aiglon soft paraffins ("VA"), the results within a group are comparable. The artificially manufactured samples ("SW"-samples) are found to have the smallest solubility values. A correlation between the a/a ratio and the solubility was not observed.

## 4.2 Liquid and solid paraffin measurements

Liquid and hard paraffin samples contain very small amounts of MOAH compared to soft paraffin samples (Table 4), with two exceptions being the samples "SN600BO" (0.885% MOAH) and "SN600TWO" (0.158% MOAH). The first one is a dark, viscous base oil obtained after solvent dewaxing in the purification process of mineral oil products. The subsequent hydrogenation procedure decreases the amount of aromatic compounds leading to technical white oils like sample "SN600TWO", as can be seen in Table 4. According to the monograph of the Ph.Eur., liquid paraffins like Paraffinum liquidum and Paraffinum perliquidum should not contain any MOAH. Nevertheless, small amounts of MOAH could be detected for several paraffin samples (Table 4). For instance, both Paraffinum perliquidum and Paraffinum liquidum are found to have comparable values of MOAH.

The samples "OX 415", "OX 420", and "OX 430" from Shell are declared as synthetic white oils. Synthetically produced paraffin products should not contain any aromatic compounds due to the synthetic process. Indeed, no MOAH signals could be observed for these samples.

**Table 4.** Overview of the liquid and hard paraffin samples measured. The content of MOAH is displayed as an integral ratio of the respective aromatic and aliphatic parts.

| Description | Sample-ID | aromatic/aliphatic protons [%] |
| --- | --- | --- |
| Light Liquid Paraffin | Parperl1 | 0 |
| Light Liquid Paraffin | P2076 | 0 |
| Synthetic liquid paraffin | OX 415 | 0 |
| Synthetic liquid paraffin | OX 420 | 0 |
| Synthetic liquid paraffin | OX 430 | 0 |
| Liquid Paraffin | Parliq1 | 0.0005 |
| Liquid Paraffin | Parliq2 | 0.0006 |
| Light Liquid Paraffin | Parperl2 | 0.0009 |
| Liquid Paraffin | P6501 | 0.0018 |
| Liquid Paraffin | SN600MWO | 0.0024 |
| Liquid Paraffin | P2071 | 0.0036 |
| Hard Paraffin | ParDur | 0.0060 |
| Technical Liquid Paraffin | SN600TWO | 0.1575 |
| Paraffin intermediate | SN600BO | 0.8849 |

## 4.3 Comparison to other analytical methods characterizing MOSH or/and MOAH

The LC-GC-FID technique for the analysis of MOH, as reported in [13,14], separates the MOSH and MOAH fractions with LC first which are quantitatively evaluated with GC due to their retention behavior. However, this method [13,14] does not consider the whole sample for analysis because of cutting some fractions upon transition from LC to GC. Thus, compounds with specific retention behavior are disregarded. Furthermore, integration is done within certain windows, excluding components with higher or lower molecular masses. Overestimation of MOAH occurs when MOSH appear in the MOAH fraction due to their similar retention behavior. In LC-GC-MS, no information about the physicochemical properties of the compounds is available. The equipment is quite complex, special know-how for methodology and interpretation of results is required, and measurement times are pretty long. In contrast, our $^{1}$H NMR method provides a simple and fast sample preparation, only composed of diluting the sample in a solvent mixture. Processing and evaluating the spectra are simple procedures as well and can often be done automatically. Thanks to the highly selective and precise nature of NMR, MOAH protons can surely be distinguished from MOSH protons. A limitation of NMR is the low sensitivity which sometimes makes detection of traces of MOAH challenging.

The PULCON methodology used for analysis of mineral oil-based products [15] requires identical treatment for analyte and reference sample, i.e. concentration, receiver gain, excitation angle and sample volume. Thus, this method is prone to errors. The MOAH fraction was determined using naphthalene equivalents, whereas decalin was chosen as the saturated counterpart to determine the MOSH fraction [15]. Actually, there is no reference substance which is appropriate for representing an average structure of the fractions of MOSH/MOAH.

The amount of MOSH and MOAH analyzed by LC-GC-FID and PULCON methodology is given in mass percent which might be useful for direct comparisons with other methods. However, it is not practicable to directly compare our results given in a proton ratio to data that provides mass concentration.

## 5. Conclusion

The [1]H NMR method is holistic and unique for the determination of aromatic hydrocarbons in paraffins. The results are selective and precise if carried out in a validated and experienced way. The results are representing the proton ratios of the aromatic to the aliphatic chemical moieties of the paraffins and can be interpreted as the percentage of the aromatic part. From a toxicological point of view, the results are also advantageous since the aromatic protons can only result from the unsubstituted parts of an aromatic core. Steric hindrance resulting from an aliphatic substitution is recognized and decreases the result in an expected way. Moreover, by our results the refinery process could be followed with respect to residual traces of aromatic impurities. Moreover, the comparison of a lot of products on the German market was done and revealed that a sufficient refinement of the products is possible. By using synthetic products, a very high degree of purity with respect to aromatic impurities is possible. Applying our [1]H NMR method, the production process – the refinement – of the paraffins may be verified. Our future investigation will focus on the correlation of this sophisticated analytical method with simpler UV analytics of the aromatic component. The results doubtless show that the content of aromatic components in paraffins for pharmaceutical use is very low compared to the daily intake by food and environmental pollution.

# References

[1] American Petroleum Institute (API), Selected values of properties of hydrocarbons and related compounds, Research Project 44, Department of Chemistry, Agricultural and Mechanical College of Texas, TX, USA, 1961.

[2] R. Agarwal, S. Kumar, N.K. Mehrotra, Polyaromatic Hydrocarbon Profile of a Mineral Oil (JBO-P) by Gas Chromatography. Journal of Chromatographic Science. 24 (1986) 289-292.

[3] Council of Europe, paraffin, light liquid monograph No. 07/2018: 0240, in: European Pharmacopeia, 9th ed., Strasbourg, 2018, p. 5737.

[4] Council of Europe, paraffin, liquid monograph No. 07/2018:0239, in: European Pharmacopeia, 9th ed., Strasbourg, 2018, pp. 5737-5738.

[5] Council of Europe, paraffin, hard monograph No. 01/2008:1034, in: European Pharmacopeia, 9th ed., Strasbourg, 2018, pp. 3268-3269.

[6] United States Pharmacopeial Convention, United States Pharmacopeia, 29th ed., Rockville, 2006.

[7] Council of Europe, paraffin, white soft monograph No. 07/2009:1799, in: European Pharmacopeia, 9th ed., Strasbourg, 2018, pp. 3270-3271.

[8] Council of Europe, paraffin, yellow soft monograph No. 07/2008:1554, corrected 6.8, in: European Pharmacopeia, 9th ed., Strasbourg, 2018, p. 3271.

[9] A. Sarkman, Arzneibuch-Kommentar, Wissenschaftliche Verlagsgesellschaft Stuttgart, Stuttgart, Govi-Verlag – Pharmazeutischer Verlag GmbH, Eschborn, 58. Aktualisierungslieferung, 2018.

[10] J.G. Speight, The chemistry and technology of petroleum, third ed., CRC Press, Boca Raton, 2006.

[11] European Food Safety Authority (EFSA, Scientific opinion on Mineral Oil Hydrocarbons in Food, EFSA Journal. 10 (2012) 4-5.

[12] G.R. Blackburn, R.A. Deitch, C.A. Schreiner et al., Estimation of the dermal carcinogenic activity of petroleum fractions using a modified Ames assay, Cell Biology and Toxicology. 1 (1984) 67-80.

[13] K. Grob, M. Biedermann, A. Caramaschi et al., LC-GC Analysis of the Aromatics in a Mineral Oil Fraction: Batching Oil for Jute Bags, Journal of High Resolution Chromatography. 14 (1991) 33-39.

[14] M. Biedermann, K. Grob, On-line coupled high performance liquid chromatography-gas chromatography for the analysis of contamination by mineral oil. Part 1: Method of analysis, Journal of Chromatography A. 1255 (2012) 56-75.

[15] D. Lachenmeier, G. Mildau, A. Rullmann et al., Evaluation of mineral oil saturated hydrocarbons (MOSH) and mineral oil aromatic hydrocarbons (MOAH) in pure mineral hydrocarbon-based cosmetics raw materials using [1]H NMR spectroscopy, F1000 Research. 6 (2017) 682.

[16] U. Holzgrabe, Quantitative NMR spectroscopy in pharmaceutical applications, Progress in Nuclear Magnetic Resonance Spectroscopy. 57 (2010) 229-240.

[17] ICH Guideline Q2 (R1) Validation of Analytical Procedures: Text and Methodology. 1996, Geneva, Switzerland. Available from: <http://www.ich.org/products/guidelines/quality/quality-single/article/validation-of-analytical-procedures-text-and-methodology.html>.

[18] E. Pretsch, P. Bühlmann, C. Affolter, M. Badertscher, Spektroskopische Daten zur Strukturaufklärung organischer Verbindungen, 4th ed.,Springer, Berlin, 2001.

## 6. Correspondance Letter

Lachenmeier et al. commented in a correspondence letter [1] on the publication presented in section 3.1.1, where requirements for the accurate analysis of MOH using NMR spectroscopy were pointed out. The main statements are listed in the following.

- Selection of integration windows: the region from $\delta$ = 3.0 - 4.0 ppm does not reflect MOSH signals but rather non-aliphatic compounds, leading to overestimation of MOSH. The residual water signal and the $^{13}C$ satellites of $CHCl_3$ should be excluded from integration to avoid overestimation of MOAH.
- The PULCON methodology is appropriate for the quantification of MOAH and MOSH in paraffins for medicinal and cosmetic use.
- Absolute quantification of MOAH is superior to the calculation of the MOAH/MOSH ratio.

The reply is given in the companion paper

**Reply to "Requirements for accurate [1]H NMR quantification of mineral oil hydrocarbons (paraffins) for pharmaceutical or cosmetic use"**

<u>Jonas Urlaub</u>, Jochen Norwig, Curd Schollmayer, Ulrike Holzgrabe

Reprinted with permission from J. Pharm. Biomed. Anal. 2019, 171, 235-237.

Copyright (2019) Elsevier.

The aim of our study was to design a simple and very robust method [2], which can be used on a routine NMR machine from 400 MHz onwards [3,4], because the philosophy of the European Pharmacopoeia is to establish methods, which do not need any extra tools. In addition, the European Pharmacopoeia does not want to rely on one producer of a machine, further software or SOPs. Thus, the food screener used for PULCON (Pulse length based concentration determination) does not meet this requirement and is not available in each quality assessment laboratory of regulatory authorities (e.g. BfArM or EDQM) and pharmaceutical industry environment. The usage of PULCON requires to consider machine specific characteristics and is not applicable to other machines without comprehensive adjustments. Moreover, PULCON, which was originally developed for the determination of protein content [e.g. 5], is nowadays mainly used in food chemistry. The number of applications using PULCON in the field of drug analysis is very limited, moreover the number of papers dealing with PULCON is also low. In SCifinder and Pubmed less than 20 papers can be found only.

In our paper [2] we presented a method that can be much easier validated in routine analysis. We do not even need any standard, since the sample itself provides the necessary information with all the advantages of an internal standard. In contrast, PULCON is a qNMR methodology using an external standard. The NMR tubes must have a constant active sample volume of the individual samples. This means sample tubes with very good specifications must be used and/or a correction factor must be determined for each tube. The sensitivity of the NMR coil must be corrected for each sample. Therefore, the probe must be tuned and matched accordingly and the actual pulse length for every sample must be known [6]. An error in pulse length is more critical when using a 30° pulse for acquisition than a 90° pulse. Hence, a 90° pulse might be a better choice. However, the relaxation time will be longer and along with this the analysis time [6,7].

It is correct and necessary to take residual solvent signals (and their $^{13}$C satellites, eventually) into consideration for correct qNMR measurement [8,9]. However, integrating the residual solvent signal of $H_2O$ does not lead to significant deviations of our results. The MOSH integral is quite large and thus the $H_2O$ signal has small influence, especially when determining the MOAH/MOSH ratio (cf. Table 1). The $^{13}$C satellites of $CHCl_3$ do not significantly influence the MOAH/MOSH ratio either (cf. Fig. 1a), especially when using a $CDCl_3$ solvent with a high degree of deuteration (99.96 atom %). Thus, we decided not to use $^{13}$C decoupling. Decoupling during acquisition leads to heating effects of sample and probe due to the additional radiation of radio frequency. This requires a reduction of the acquisition time. Consequently, digital resolution will be less and truncation effects will occur. In our opinion, the pretty small influence of the $^{13}$C satellites on the MOAH/MOSH ratio does not justify the effort of selective decoupling experiments.

Mineral oil hydrocarbons (MOH) are a very complex mixture of different substances. Using [1]H NMR spectroscopy, there is no complete resolution of proton signals within the MOSH region, so the question arises if the integration window of $\delta = 3.0 - 0.2$ ppm as suggested by Lachenmeier et al. [10] is appropriate. Cutting the integration window at $\delta = 3.0$ ppm carries the risk of disregarding protons of $CH_2$ groups attached to polycyclic aromatic hydrocarbons (PAH) [11]. Actually, integrating the MOSH protons from $\delta = 3.0 - 0.2$ ppm (Fig. 1) results in a deviation of + 0.14% compared to our MOAH/MOSH results where the integration window from $\delta = 4.0 - 0.16$ ppm was applied (data not shown). This is not considered significant.

A normalization method is useful in the case a multicomponent system has to be characterized and the quantity of each component is of interest, e.g. in the case of gentamicin consisting of at least 5 components [12-14]. Here, we just want to determine the MOAH/MOSH ratio, thus considering the two integrals of MOSH and MOAH, only. The results of normalization and ratio establishment are not significantly different. This can be seen in Table 1. Hence, the regulatory authorities can decide whether they want to define either the ratio or the normalization as a requirement. Concerning our acquisition parameters, we used a spectral width of 30 ppm (pulse length: 9 µs) to facilitate appropriate phasing and baseline correction. A digital resolution of at least 0.2 Hz was ensured. The signal-to-noise ratio was not significantly influenced by increasing the acquisition time of the FID. We decided to use 256 scans since this procedure resulted in a good compromise between analysis time and signal-to-noise ratio even for samples with small amounts of MOAH.

**Table 1.** Results of normalization and ratio establishment for the determination of MOAH in some representative samples.

| Sample | MOAH/MOSH ratio in percent | MOAH/MOH ratio in percent (Normalization) | MOAH/MOSH ratio in percent ($H_2O$ signal excluded) |
|---|---|---|---|
| CJUS | 0.067 | 0.067 | 0.068 |
| F | 0.215 | 0.214 | 0.217 |
| C2 | 0.490 | 0.488 | 0.492 |
| TV1 | 0.383 | 0.382 | 0.385 |
| VasFlav | 0.477 | 0.475 | 0.480 |

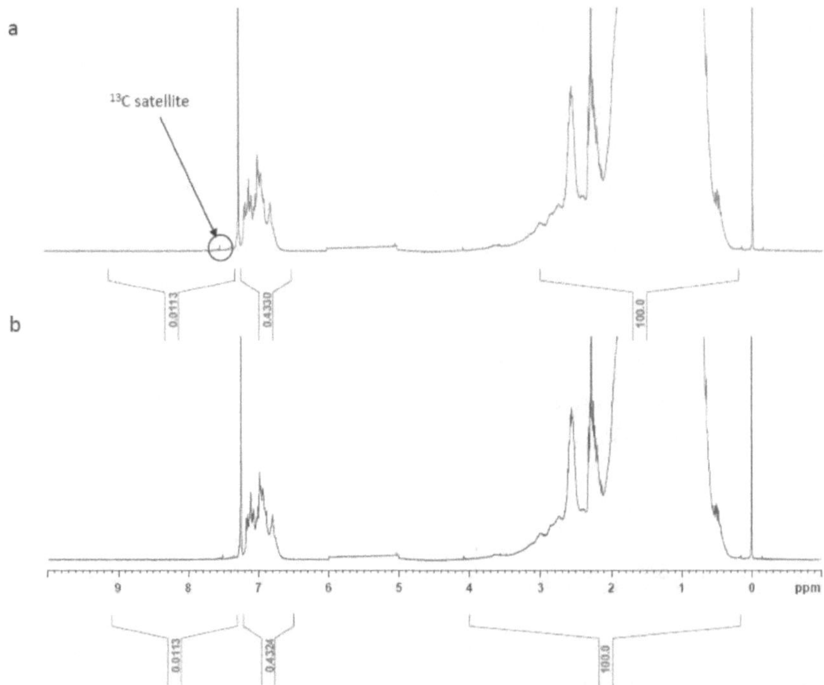

**Figure 1.** $^1$H NMR spectra of the soft paraffin sample „D". MOSH region integrated from δ = 0.2 - 3.0 ppm (a) and from δ = 0.16 - 4.0 ppm (b). The integral of the $^{13}$C satellite marked in (a) is 0.0010 related to the MOSH integral (not shown).

Lachenmeier et al. claimed that we misinterpreted the monographs of liquid paraffins like paraffinum liquidum and paraffinum perliquidum in the Ph.Eur. as we said that these products should not contain any MOAH. However, the Ph.Eur. limits the PAH by the UV method (after DMSO extraction). Indeed, liquid paraffins meet the specification of the Ph.Eur. even if they contain small amounts of MOAH. According to the commentary to the monograph of liquid paraffin of the Ph.Eur. [15], unsaturated and aromatic MOH have to be removed from the final product. Furthermore, it is supposed by Lachenmeier et al. to consider naphthalene and decalin equivalents for the interpretation of our results. Neither naphthalene nor decalin (i.e. decahydronaphthalene) are appropriate for a variety of reasons. Basically, they represent the polyaromatic hydrocarbons (PAHs) only, but the toxic components to be limited are a mixture of PAHs substituted with hydrocarbon chains of different length and branching grade, summarized as MOAH. We did not want to simply replace the insufficient UV method, providing an artificial value, with an equivalent method. We wanted to establish a method, which provides more information due to the toxicity discussions regarding paraffins and corresponding products. Hence, it makes no sense to consider naphthalene and decalin equivalents for interpretation. Furthermore, using equivalents in this particular analysis problem is a risky approach, since we do not exactly know the molecular masses of the analytes.

## References

[1] J. Geisser, J. Teipel, T. Kuballa, S. Weber, G. Mildau, S. Walch, D. Lachenmeier, Requirements for accurate [1]H NMR quantification of mineral oil hydrocarbons (paraffins) for pharmaceutical use, J. Pharm. Biomed. Anal. 171 (2019) 232-234.

[2] J. Urlaub, J. Norwig, C. Schollmayer, U. Holzgrabe, [1]H NMR analytical characterization of mineral oil hydrocarbons (PARAFFINS) for pharmaceutical use, J. Pharm. Biomed. Anal. 169 (2019) 41-48.

[3] Council of Europe, Heparin sodium monograph No. 01/2018:0333, in: European Pharmacopoeia, 9th ed., 2018, pp. 4913-4915, Strasbourg.

[4] T. Beyer, B. Diehl, G. Randel, E. Humpfner, H. Schäfer, M. Spraul, C. Schollmayer, U. Holzgrabe, Quality assessment of unfractionated heparin using [1]H nuclear magnetic resonance spectroscopy, J. Pharm. Biomed. Anal. 48 (2008) 13-19.

[5] G. Wider, L. Dreier, Measuring Protein Concentrations by NMR Spectroscopy, J. Am. Chem. Soc. 128 (2006) 2571-2576.

[6] T. Claridge, High-Resolution NMR Techniques in Organic Chemistry, 3rd ed., Elsevier, Amsterdam, 2016.

[7] T. Kühn (VP Applications Development, Bruker Biospin GmbH), qNMR und Reinheitsbestimmung, Bruker BioSpin NMR User Meeting Karlsruhe (2016).

[8] U. Holzgrabe, Quantitative NMR spectroscopy in pharmaceutical applications, Prog. Nucl. Magn. Reson. Spectrosc. 57 (2010) 229-240.

[9] U. Holzgrabe, Magnetic Resonance: Quantitative NMR – method and applications, in: J.C. Lindon (Ed.), Encyclopedia of Spectroscopy and Spectrometry, 2nd ed., Elsevier, Kidlington, Oxford, UK, 2010, pp. 2331-2339.

[10] D. Lachenmeier, G. Mildau, A. Krause, G. Marx, S. G. Walch, A. Hartwig, T. Kuballa, Evaluation of mineral oil saturated hydrocarbons (MOSH) and mineral oil aromatic hydrocarbons (MOAH) in pure mineral hydrocarbon-based cosmetics raw materials using [1]H NMR spectroscopy, F1000 Res. 6 (2017) 682.

[11] S. Bienz, L. Bigler, T. Fox, H. Meier, Spektroskopische Methoden in der organischen Chemie, 9th ed., Thieme, Stuttgart, 2016.

[12] Council of Europe, Gentamicin sulfate monograph No. 07/2012:0331 corrected 7.6, in: European Pharmacopoeia, 9th ed., 2018, pp. 2573-2574, Strasbourg.

[13] F. Wienen, R. Deubner, U. Holzgrabe, Composition and impurity profile of multisource raw material of gentamicin - a comparison, Pharmeuropa 15 (2003) 273-279.

[14] R. Deubner, U. Holzgrabe, Micellar electrokinetic capillary chromatography, high performance liquid chromatography and nuclear magnetic resonance – three orthogonal methods for characterization of critical drugs, J. Pharm. Biomed. Anal. 35 (2004) 459-467.

[15] A. Sarkman, Dickflüssiges Paraffin No. 05/0239, in: Arzneibuch-Kommentar, Wissenschaftliche Verlagsgesellschaft Stuttgart, Stuttgart, Govi-Verlag – Pharmazeutischer Verlag GmbH, Eschborn, 54. Aktualisierungslieferung, 2016.

## 3.1.2 Evaluation of MOAH in pharmaceutical paraffins by $^1$H NMR spectroscopy without sample solvent

### 1. Introduction

In $^1$H NMR spectroscopy, the analyte is usually dissolved in a deuterated solvent to avoid signal distortion caused by the solute protons. However, residual $^1$H nuclei in deuterated solvents and proton-deuterium exchanges taking place inside the sample solution lead to characteristic residual solvent signals, which might overlap with the signals of the analyte [1]. Additionally, it must be taken into account that deuterated solvents such as chloroform-d or DMSO-$d_6$ are likely to contain residual water and other dissolved impurities which might interfere with sample signals as well. Whereas the latter is mainly dependent on the quality of the solvent, the problem of residual solvent signals can be addressed by applying certain pulse sequences, the solvent suppression techniques. A huge toolbox of such techniques is available, which are widely employed for the suppression of the water signal because it is a frequently used solvent in bioanalytical chemistry [2,3], but also for the suppression of other residual solvent signals [4]. However, complications such as incomplete solvent suppression, attenuation of the covered analyte protons or phase and/or baseline distortions might arise if resonances under or near the solvent signal are of main interest [5,6].

For the evaluation of the mineral oil aromatic hydrocarbons (MOAH) and mineral oil saturated hydrocarbons (MOSH) in paraffins for pharmaceutical use, a $^1$H NMR spectroscopy method was applied in chapter 3.1.1 using CDCl$_3$ as sample solvent. For the evaluation of the aromatic/aliphatic ratio, abbreviated as a/a ratio in the following, of the paraffin samples, the residual solvent signal of CHCl$_3$ within the MOAH region was excluded from integration, whereas the water signal (originating from the CDCl$_3$ solvent) was included for integration. Here, a simple alternative to the artificially removed solvent signal applying special pulsing techniques was considered for the paraffin sample measurement. Overlapping of the residual solvent resonances, its residual water and potential impurities with the analyte protons was avoided by preparing the paraffin sample without solvent, which was measured by means of $^1$H NMR spectroscopy afterwards. The approach was tested on a soft paraffin sample which was already measured by the $^1$H NMR spectroscopic method described in chapter 3.1.1. The calculated a/a ratio was then compared to the results obtained in chapter 3.1.1.

# 2. Experimental section

## 2.1 Samples and chemicals

The soft paraffin sample (Sample D) was provided by Sasol Wax (Hamburg, Germany). Deuteriumoxide ($D_2O \geq 99.9$ atom % D containing 0.05 wt. % 3-(trimethylsilyl)propionic-2,2,3,3-$d_4$ acid, sodium salt, TSP) by Sigma-Aldrich Chemie GmbH (Steinheim, Germany). The coaxial tubes and respective inserts were purchased from Deutero GmbH (Kastellaun, Germany).

## 2.2 Sample preparation

A 1 mL syringe was filled with the soft paraffin sample, then approximately 500 µL were injected into the coaxial tube, which was meanwhile placed inside a water bath at 80 °C to facilitate the sample transfer. The insert was filled with 200 µL $D_2O$ (for generating the lock signal), which contained 0.05 wt. % TSP, and placed inside the tube.

## 2.3 Sample measurement

The measurements were conducted on a Bruker Avance III 400 MHz UltraShield instrument with a 5-mm PABBI ATM 1 H/D-BB Z-GRD probehead, a Bruker automatic sample changer (B-ACS 60), a BSVT (Bruker Smart Variable Temperature System), and a BCU05 (Bruker Cooling Unit). The temperature during measurements was maintained at 300 K and 340 K, respectively. The $^1$H NMR spectra recording was performed as described in chapter 3.1.1 using the baseopt mode (Bruker standard zg pulse sequence) with a pulse angle of 90° and 256 scans. The spectral width was 30 ppm and the size of the FID (TD) was 128k. The acquisition time was 5.45 s and the relaxation delay (D1) was 10 s. All measurements were performed without rotation. The chemical shifts were referred to the TSP signal at $\delta = 0$ ppm. All spectra were processed using the TopSpin 4.0.2 software by Bruker (Bruker BioSpin, Rheinstetten, Germany). Both phase correction (0. and 1. order) and integration were performed manually. The baseline correction was performed from $\delta = -2 - 5$ ppm

(MOSH region) and from $\delta = 6 - 10$ ppm (MOAH region). The a/a ratio was calculated by dividing the MOAH through the MOSH integral.

## 3. Results and discussion

$D_2O$ was favored as the deuterated lock solvent because it combines the advantages of a high boiling point (101 °C) and showing no residual solvent signals in the spectral areas of interest. Before sample measurement, the relaxation delay (D1) was checked to be sufficient to provide full relaxation of the MOAH and MOSH protons using the inversion recovery experiment. $^1$H NMR spectra of the soft paraffin sample measured at three temperatures (300, 313 and 340 K) with and without using sample solvent are shown in Fig. 1A-C (MOAH region) and 2A-C (MOSH region). As can be seen, the spectra in Fig. 1A and B only slightly differ in chemical shift and resolution.

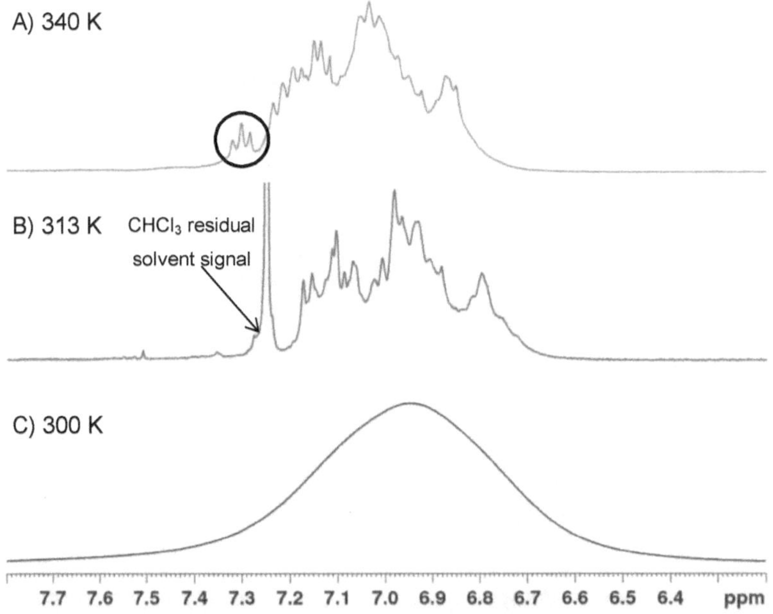


**Figure 1.** Expanded part of the $^1$H NMR spectra of Sample D ($\delta = 6.2 - 7.8$ ppm, MOAH region), measured at three different temperatures. A) 340 K; coaxial tube with insert ($D_2O$), no sample solvent used; B) 313 K; 25 mg/mL paraffin sample dissolved in CDCl$_3$; C) 300 K; coaxial tube with insert ($D_2O$), no sample solvent used.

The MOAH protons reveal a triplet like signal pattern at about δ = 7.3 ppm (Fig. 1A, circled) which is covered by the residual solvent signal at δ = 7.25 ppm in Fig. 1B. In contrast, no signal pattern within the MOAH region could be observed at 300 K (Fig. 1C) due to massive line broadening, merely forming a hump of unresolved signals. This is caused by the extremely limited movement of analyte molecules, resulting from low temperatures or high viscosity [6].

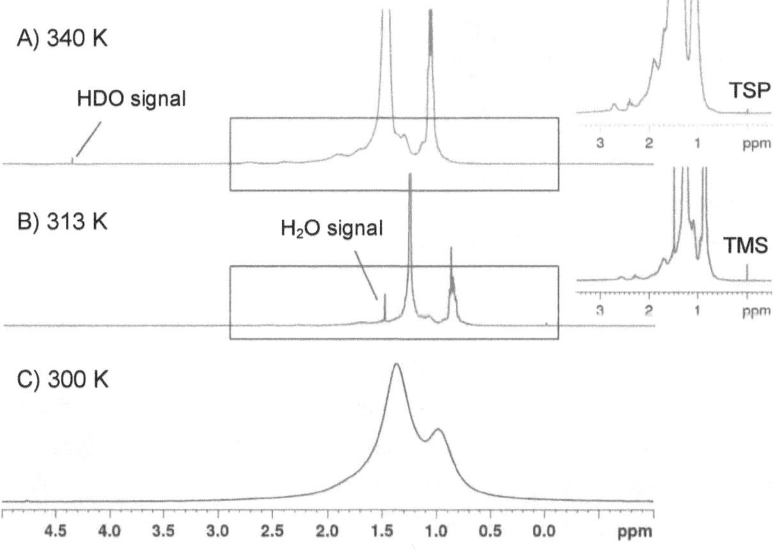


**Figure 2.** $^1$H NMR spectra of Sample D (MOSH region) measured at different temperatures applying different sample preparations. A) 340 K; coaxial tube with insert (D$_2$O), no sample solvent used. B) 313 K; 25 mg/mL paraffin sample dissolved in CDCl$_3$. C) 300 K; coaxial tube with insert (D$_2$O), no sample solvent used. Enlarged spectral regions are shown at the right of the respective spectrum. Reference standards: TMS (tetramethylsilane), TSP (3-(trimethylsilyl)propionic-2,2,3,3-d$_4$ acid, sodium salt).

Similar observations were made for the MOSH protons (Fig. 2A-C). Of course, the residual water signal at δ = 1.5 ppm disappeared when no sample solvent was used (Fig. 2A and C). When the insert with D$_2$O was applied, the HDO signal arose at δ = 4.5 ppm, which was not overlapping with signals of interest though (Fig. 2A).

Tab. 1 shows an overview of the a/a ratio results, obtained from different integration approaches. The a/a ratio measured at 313 K was 0.4437, excluding the $CHCl_3$ signal at δ = 7.25 ppm (chapter 3.1.1). Here, the water signal at δ = 1.5 ppm within the MOSH region was not excluded from integration because it was assumed being neglectable as part of the tremendous integral of the MOSH.

**Table 1.** Overview of the resulting a/a ratios of Sample D.

| | Sample D (soft paraffin) | | |
| --- | --- | --- | --- |
| | 300 K (no solvent) | 313 K (CDCl$_3$) | 340 K (no solvent) |
| | | 0.4437[d] | |
| a/a ratio | | 0.4472[b] | 0.4478[b] |
| | 0.4694[a] | 0.4665[c] | 0.4672[a] |

a) Integration without exclusions

b) Integration excluding the $CHCl_3$ and water signal (313 K)

c) Integration considering the area below the $CHCl_3$ signal and the water signal (313 K)

d) see chapter 3.1.1.

As a first approach to compare the a/a ratio results, the water signal within the MOSH region (Fig. 2B) was considered by excluding the protruding part of the signal, resulting in an a/a ratio of 0.4472 (increase of 0.8%, Tab. 1). This was in good accordance with the results obtained at 340 K (0.4478). For the ensuing approach, the area covered by the $CHCl_3$ signal (Fig. 1B) was considered by adding to the MOAH integral obtained by the aforementioned integration procedure (a/a = 0.4472). This was achieved by calculating the percentage amount of the respective area within the MOAH region (circled in Fig. 1A), resulting in 4.3%. The area for integration was determined by overlaying the both spectra (Fig. 1A and B). Assuming the $CHCl_3$ residual solvent signal to cover 4.3% of the MOAH fraction, the corrected a/a ratio was calculated, resulting in 0.4665, which is in good accordance with the a/a ratios obtained at 300 K (0.4696) and 340 K (0.4672).

Although calculations of the a/a ratios do not require sufficient resolution of the MOAH and MOSH signals, the broad lines obtained at 300 K (Fig. 1C and 2C) complicated phasing and integration procedures. Hence, appropriate evaluation of results was unfeasible. Elevating the temperature to 340 K significantly reduced these complications (Fig. 2A). For the corrected a/a calculations and comparisons of the spectra, the "true" a/a ratio was assumed not to be influenced by temperature or sample preparation which was justified by the chemical indifference of white soft paraffin [7].

## 4. Conclusion

It could be demonstrated that $^1$H NMR measurements performed without sample solvent are appropriate for the evaluation of the a/a ratio in soft paraffin. The results are in good accordance with the previously yielded in chapter 3.1.1, when the area under the $CHCl_3$ residual solvent signal is considered. The rather unconventional approach described in this study is advantageous because there are no interfering residual solvent signals. However, the sample preparation is more elaborate.

## 5. References

[1] A.E. Derome, Modern NMR Techniques for Chemistry Research. Pergamon Press, Oxford, 1987.

[2] M. Guéron, P. Plateau, M. Decorps, Solvent signal suppression in NMR. Progr. Nucl. Magn. Reson. Spectrosc. 1991, 23, 135-209.

[3] W.S. Price, Water signal suppression in NMR spectroscopy. Annu. Rep. NMR Spectrosc. 1999, 38, 289-354.

[4] T. Venâncio, L.A. Colnago, Improvements in the CWFP method for solvent suppression in high resolution NMR, 12th nuclear magnetic resonance users meeting, 3rd iberoamerican NMR meeting 2009, Extended Abstracts Book 2009, pp. 77-78.

[5] M. Liu, X.A. Mao, C. Ye, H. Huang, J.K. Nicholson, J.C. Lindon, Improved WATERGATE Pulse Sequences for Solvent Suppression in NMR Spectroscopy. J. Magn. Reson. 1998, 132, 125-129.

[6] O. Zerbe, S. Jurt, Applied NMR Spectroscopy for Chemists and Life Scientists. Wiley-VCH, Weinheim, 2014.

[7] Kommentar zum Europäischen Arzneibuch, Monographie 8.0/1799 – Weißes Vaselin. 52. Aktualisierungslieferung, Wissenschaftliche Verlagsgesellschaft Stuttgart, Stuttgart, 2015.

## 3.1.3 Characterization of paraffins: comparison of $^1$H NMR and UV/Vis spectroscopic data

### 1. Introduction

Paraffins are mineral oil derived mixtures of structurally differing hydrocarbons, which are generally referred to as mineral oil hydrocarbons (MOH) [1]. The MOH can be divided into the mineral oil saturated hydrocarbons (MOSH) and mineral oil aromatic hydrocarbons (MOAH). The MOAH may contain mono- and polycyclic aromatic hydrocarbons, referred to as MAH and PAH, respectively. The latter may exhibit allergenic and carcinogenic potential and are thus limited by purity tests in the latest compendial monographs of paraffins for pharmaceutical use [2,3,4].

The purity assessment of paraffins within the Pharmacopoeias has been altered over time. In the German Pharmacopoeia (Deutsches Arzneibuch 8, DAB 8), a UV test was implemented to support the sulfuric acid test (test for the extent of paraffin refining), because the latter was considered less specific and robust with respect to the determination of the PAH [5].

The UV test of the DAB 8 is based on the assumption that the UV/Vis spectra of paraffins are indicative of their relative content of MOAH [5,6]. The amounts of MAH and PAH in soft, liquid and solid paraffins were limited by the absorbances at the three wavelengths $\lambda = 275$, 295 nm and $\lambda > 300$ nm, which should not exceed prescribed thresholds [7-10]. The rough assignment of MOAH with one (MAH), two, and three or more aromatic rings (PAH) to $\lambda = 275$, 295 nm, and $\lambda > 300$ nm is referred to the UV/Vis spectra of benzene, naphthalene and other polycondensed aromatic compounds, taking into account the bathochromic shift caused by the alkyl substituents [11]. An overview of the compendial tests according to DAB 8 is given in Tab. 1.

In the subsequent editions of the DAB and in the Ph.Eur., the UV test was replaced by another method employing UV/Vis spectroscopy, which was described by the Food and Drug Administration (FDA) [12,13]. Here, the absorbance of the DMSO extract of a paraffin sample was determined from $\lambda = 260 - 420$ nm, which was compared to a naphthalene reference solution measured at $\lambda = 275$ nm. This approach provides a more specific and sensitive detection of the carcinogenic PAH compared to the UV method of the DAB 8 (detection limit = 0.2 and 1.0 ppm, respectively) [5,12]. However, the test considers the amount of PAH alone instead of the entire MOAH fraction.

As stated above, the UV/Vis spectra of paraffins can support the evaluation of MOAH because they roughly reflect the quantity of aromatic compounds. In chapter 3.1.1, it has been shown that NMR spectroscopy is also capable of determining the MOAH content in paraffin samples based on the MOAH/MOSH ratio. A study concerned with the comparison of UV and NMR spectroscopic determination of MOAH in paraffins has not been reported yet. For this purpose, the UV tests according to DAB 8 were performed on the majority of the paraffin samples analyzed in chapter 3.1.1. The UV results and the aromatic/aliphatic ratios obtained from [1]H NMR measurements were tested for linear correlation, which was supplemented by the evaluation of the UV/Vis and [1]H NMR spectra of representative paraffin samples.

**Table 1.** UV tests for purity evaluation of paraffins according to DAB 8. *l*: optical path length.

| | Soft paraffins [7] | | Liquid paraffins [8,9] | | Solid paraffins [10] |
|---|---|---|---|---|---|
| **Test** | a) | b) | a) | b) | |
| **Sample** | 0.50 g/50 mL | 1:10 dilution of solution a) | Crude substance | Crude substance | 0.50 g/50 mL |
| **Solvent** | Isooctane | Isooctane | none | none | Isooctane |
| **l (cm)** | 0.5 | 2.0 | 0.5 | 2.0 | 2.0 |
| **Absorbance limits** | 0.60 (> 300 nm) | 0.80 (275 nm) 0.40 (295 nm) | 0.80 (275 nm) | 0.40 (295 nm) 0.30 (> 300 nm) | 0.60 (275 nm) 0.30 (295 nm) 0.10 (> 310 nm) |
| **Reference** | Isooctane | Isooctane | Water | Water | Isooctane |

## 2. Experimental section

### 2.1 Materials and methods

### 2.1.1 Chemicals and reagents

Isooctane of analytical grade was purchased from Merck KGaA (Darmstadt, Germany) and VWR international (Leuven, Belgium). A total of 47 paraffin samples were analyzed by UV spectroscopy, including 34 soft paraffins, 11 liquid paraffins, one solid paraffin and one paraffin intermediate. The samples have already been characterized by means of $^1$H NMR spectroscopy, which is comprehensively described in chapter 3.1.1.

### 2.1.2 Apparatus and equipment

The UV/Vis spectroscopic measurements were performed on a Uvikon XL spectrophotometer (BioTek Instruments, Bad Friedrichshall, Germany) and a Varian Cary 50 Bio spectrophotometer (Varian Inc, part of Agilent Technologies, Waldbronn, Germany). For all measurements, fused silica cuvettes of 1.0 cm diameter were used.

### 2.1.2 UV spectroscopic measurements

The paraffin samples were analyzed according to DAB 8 by the methods detailed in Tab. 1. The tests for soft paraffins were also used for the yellow soft paraffin sample (sample 35), although a monograph for yellow soft paraffin does not exist in the DAB 8. For the determination of the absorbance at $\lambda > 300$ nm, the UV spectra of the paraffin samples were recorded from $\lambda = 300 - 420$ nm. The most intense absorbance in this spectral range was used for evaluation. The measurements were conducted (n = 1) by the Federal Institute for Drugs and Medical Devices (BfArM, Bonn, Germany).

In addition, the UV/Vis spectra of three soft paraffin samples 9, 11 and 20 were recorded (low, medium and high amount of MAOH, based on $^1$H NMR results, see chapter 3.1.1). The test solutions were prepared by dissolving varying amounts of the respective paraffin sample in isooctane. If necessary, the mixture was slightly heated up to about 50 °C to facilitate dissolution and allowed to cool to room temperature (approx. 22 °C) prior to measurement. The sample concentrations were adjusted to

20 mg/mL (sample 9), 6.25 mg/mL (sample 11) and 0.64 mg/mL (sample 20), respectively, in order to obtain applicable absorption maxima of the samples, ranging from 0.6 to 0.8. The UV/Vis spectra were recorded from $\lambda$ = 200 - 500 nm with a scan speed of 600 nm/min and a scan interval of 1 nm. The blank spectrum was recorded using isooctane.

## 2.1.3 Processing and evaluation of UV and NMR data

In the $^{1}$H NMR spectra, spectral regions for the mono- and polyaromatic MOH were defined. Integration of the MOAH signals was performed between $\delta$ = 6.5 - 9.1 ppm. For the soft and solid paraffins, the $CHCl_3$ residual solvent signal from $\delta$ = 7.22 - 7.3 ppm was excluded from integration. The signals of the PAH were integrated between $\delta$ = 7.3 - 9.1 ppm, the signals of the MAH between $\delta$ = 6.5 - 7.3 ppm for liquid paraffins and between $\delta$ = 6.5 - 7.22 ppm for soft and solid paraffins. Similar spectral regions were suggested by Weber et al. [14]. The assignment of MOH to the spectral regions is summarized in Tab. 2.

The amount of MOAH, PAH and MAH of the paraffin samples were represented by the MOAH/MOSH, PAH/MOSH and MAH/MOSH ratios by setting the MOAH, PAH and MAH protons in relation to the MOSH protons ($\delta$ = 0.16 - 4 ppm) in the $^{1}$H NMR spectrum as performed in chapter 3.1.1.

**Table 2.** Assignment of MOAH, PAH and MAH to the spectral regions of the $^{1}$H NMR spectra.

| Compound | MOAH | PAH | MAH |
| --- | --- | --- | --- |
| **Soft/solid paraffins** | 7.3 - 9.1 ppm<br>6.5 - 7.22 ppm | 7.3 - 9.1 ppm | 6.5 - 7.22 ppm |
| **Liquid paraffins** | 6.5 - 9.1 ppm | 7.3 - 9.1 ppm | 6.5 - 7.3 ppm |

MAH, monocyclic aromatic hydrocarbons; MOAH, mineral oil aromatic hydrocarbons; PAH, polycyclic aromatic hydrocarbons.

For statistical analysis, the UV absorbances and the aromatic/aliphatic ratios from NMR measurements were compared by applying two different correlation models, which are described in the following. For all models applied, the correlation between UV and NMR data was assumed to be linear.

First, a Spearman's rank correlation was performed on the UV absorbances at $\lambda = 275$ nm and the MOAH/MOSH ratios of various paraffin samples. The UV and $^1$H NMR spectroscopic values were transformed into ranks of ascending order, respectively (high values represent small ranks). Subsequently, the ranks of the absorbances at $\lambda = 275$ nm were plotted against the ranks of the MOAH/MOSH ratios. The strength of the relationship between the ranks was determined by calculating the Spearman's rank correlation coefficient $r_s$.

Second, a linear regression model was applied on the UV and NMR data by plotting the absorbances at $\lambda = 275$, 295 and > 300 nm against the MOAH/MOSH, PAH/MOSH or MAH/MOSH ratios, respectively. The extent of linear correlation between those data was established by calculating the coefficient of determination $R^2$. The correlations were tested for significance using a two-sided $t$-test ($\alpha = 0.05$) [15,16].

## 3. Results and discussion

According to DAB 8, for the UV purity test of paraffins, mathematical correction for deviation from the cuvette thickness is not allowed [17]. However, the use of a cuvette of a different optical path length (1.0 cm instead of 0.5 and 2.0 cm, dependent on the test) for all measurements performed in this study is considered acceptable, because the objective was to evaluate differences between the paraffin samples. The UV and $^1$H NMR measurement results are shown in Tab. 3. One soft paraffin sample "18" showed an absorbance of $\sim 3.4$ at $\lambda = 275$ nm, which was withdrawn from correlation experiments because absorbances > 2.0 should be avoided for quantitative UV analysis [18].

Of note, aromatic paraffin additives such as antioxidants can be present in the paraffin samples and may resonate or absorb in the aromatic regions of the $^1$H NMR and UV/Vis spectra, respectively. However, they cannot be selectively distinguished from MOAH in the $^1$H NMR and the UV spectra.

Characterization of paraffins: comparison of $^1$H NMR and UV/Vis spectroscopic data

**Table 3.** UV and NMR spectroscopic measurement results (n = 1). A: absorbance.

| Soft paraffins | | | | | | | |
|---|---|---|---|---|---|---|---|
| UV | | | | $^1$H NMR | | | |
| Sample No. | A (275 nm) | Rank | A (295 nm) | A (> 300 nm) | PAH/MOSH | MAH/MOSH | MOAH/MOSH | Rank |
| 1 | 0.0498 | 37 | 0.0268 | 0.0294 | 0.0025 | 0.0503 | 0.0528 | 29 |
| 2 | 0.0506 | 36 | 0.0252 | 0.0287 | 0.0024 | 0.0514 | 0.0538 | 28 |
| 3 | 0.0524 | 35 | 0.0126 | 0.0299 | 0.0017 | 0.0656 | 0.0673 | 25 |
| 4 | 0.249 | 21 | 0.126 | 0.212 | 0.0065 | 0.0928 | 0.0993 | 20 |
| 5 | 0.2496 | 20 | 0.1266 | 0.2234 | 0.0076 | 0.0902 | 0.0978 | 21 |
| 6 | 0.245 | 22 | 0.1236 | 0.2174 | 0.0087 | 0.0887 | 0.0974 | 22 |
| 7 | 0.1542 | 30 | 0.0886 | 0.1244 | 0.0050 | 0.0698 | 0.0748 | 24 |
| 8 | 0.1266 | 32 | 0.0524 | 0.0977 | 0.0042 | 0.0727 | 0.0769 | 23 |
| 9 | 0.0254 | 43 | 0.0108 | 0.0084 | 0.0019 | 0.0213 | 0.0232 | 35 |
| 10 | 0.4018 | 16 | 0.1218 | 0.1757 | 0.0113 | 0.4324 | 0.4437 | 8 |
| 11 | 0.2052 | 23 | 0.115 | 0.1792 | 0.0092 | 0.1027 | 0.1119 | 18 |
| 12 | 0.1284 | 31 | 0.0094 | 0.0392 | 0.0034 | 0.2114 | 0.2148 | 14 |
| 13 | 0.1716 | 27 | 0.0308 | 0.1052 | 0.0044 | 0.1726 | 0.1770 | 17 |
| 14 | 0.1592 | 28 | 0.037 | 0.048 | 0.0035 | 0.2291 | 0.2326 | 11 |
| 15 | 0.2992 | 19 | 0.0912 | 0.1392 | 0.0054 | 0.3116 | 0.3170 | 10 |
| 16 | 0.0344 | 41 | 0.0198 | 0.0147 | 0.0024 | 0.0241 | 0.0265 | 33 |
| 17 | 0.0606 | 34 | 0.041 | 0.0178 | 0.0024 | 0.0243 | 0.0267 | 32 |
| 18 | 3.3966 | 1 | 1.8366 | 1.5615 | 0.2325 | 0.7563 | 0.9888 | 1 |
| 19 | 0.1814 | 26 | 0.0532 | 0.079 | 0.0023 | 0.1911 | 0.1934 | 15 |
| 20 | 1.7072 | 2 | 0.8986 | 1.469 | 0.1207 | 0.6464 | 0.7671 | 2 |
| 21 | 0.6176 | 10 | 0.2572 | 0.318 | 0.0209 | 0.5273 | 0.5482 | 5 |
| 22 | 1.7022 | 3 | 0.9096 | 1.5259 | 0.1165 | 0.5691 | 0.6856 | 4 |
| 23 | 0.5834 | 11 | 0.2524 | 0.2779 | 0.0171 | 0.4727 | 0.4898 | 6 |
| 28 | 0.633 | 9 | 0.3268 | 0.4674 | 0.0408 | 0.3422 | 0.3830 | 9 |
| 29 | 0.554 | 12 | 0.345 | 0.3742 | 0.0289 | 0.1941 | 0.2230 | 12 |
| 30 | 0.4106 | 15 | 0.2462 | 0.2831 | 0.0198 | 0.1597 | 0.1795 | 16 |
| 31 | 0.0162 | 45 | 0.0022 | 0.1011 | 0.0009 | 0.0243 | 0.0252 | 34 |
| 32 | 0.0348 | 39 | 0.0096 | 0.0348 | 0.0013 | 0.0427 | 0.0440 | 31 |
| 33 | 0.0346 | 40 | 0.0078 | 0.0219 | 0.0023 | 0.0431 | 0.0454 | 30 |
| 34 | 0.1554 | 29 | 0.048 | 0.0561 | 0.0033 | 0.2122 | 0.2155 | 13 |
| 35 | 0.7244 | 6 | 0.3316 | 0.6813 | 0.0459 | 0.4311 | 0.4770 | 7 |
| 37 | 0.961 | 5 | 0.4736 | 0.8643 | 0.0883 | 0.6124 | 0.7007 | 3 |
| 38 | 0.1844 | 25 | 0.0823 | 0.1637 | 0.0078 | 0.0956 | 0.1034 | 19 |
| 39 | 0.103 | 33 | 0.0446 | 0.0277 | 0.0024 | 0.0522 | 0.0546 | 27 |
| 40 | 0.0495 | 38 | 0.0218 | 0.0325 | 0.0023 | 0.0548 | 0.0571 | 26 |

**Table 3.** (Continued)

| Liquid paraffins | | | | | | | |
|---|---|---|---|---|---|---|---|
| UV | | | | $^1$H NMR | | | |
| Sample No. | A (275 nm) | Rank | A (295 nm) | A (> 300 nm) | PAH/MOSH | MAH/MOSH | MOAH/MOSH | Rank |
| 42 | 0.1926 | 24 | 0.0864 | 0.0352 | 0 | 0 | 0 | 45 |
| 43 | 0.3232 | 18 | 0.1924 | 0.1102 | 0.0001 | 0.0008 | 0.0009 | 40 |
| 44 | 0.4211 | 14 | 0.1218 | 0.0786 | 0.0001 | 0.0004 | 0.0005 | 42 |
| 45 | 0.4419 | 13 | 0.156 | 0.0404 | 0.0001 | 0.0005 | 0.0006 | 41 |
| 46 | 1.1463 | 4 | 0.657 | 0.4304 | 0.0001 | 0.0035 | 0.0036 | 37 |
| 47 | 0.344 | 17 | 0.1232 | 0.0734 | 0 | 0 | 0 | 45 |
| 48 | 0.6974 | 7 | 0.3312 | 0.193 | 0 | 0.0018 | 0.0018 | 39 |
| 49 | 0.0077 | 47 | 0 | 0 | 0 | 0 | 0 | 45 |
| 50 | 0.0113 | 46 | 0.0236 | 0.01 | 0 | 0 | 0 | 45 |
| 51 | 0.0236 | 44 | 0.0616 | 0.0184 | 0 | 0 | 0 | 45 |
| 53 | 0.6357 | 8 | 0.2904 | 0.181 | 0.0001 | 0.0046 | 0.0024 | 38 |

| Solid paraffin | | | | | | | |
|---|---|---|---|---|---|---|---|
| Sample No. | A (275 nm) | Rank | A (295 nm) | A (> 310 nm) | PAH/MOSH | MAH/MOSH | MOAH/MOSH | Rank |
| 41 | 0.0288 | 42 | 0.0136 | 0 | 0.0014 | 0.0046 | 0.0001 | 36 |

Two assumptions were made for data evaluation: first, the $^1$H NMR spectral ranges defined in section 2.1.3 represent the PAH, MAH and the MOAH accordingly. Second, the PAH/MOSH, MAH/MOSH and MOAH/MOSH ratios are indicative for the amount of PAH, MAH and MOAH, respectively. This is based on the research performed in chapter 3.1.1, where the protons of the MOSH were used as internal standard for the determination of the amount of MOAH.

## 3.1 Rank correlation of UV and NMR data

A rank correlation including all measured paraffin samples was initially performed in order to get a rough overview of the spectroscopic data, test the validity of the assumed linear relationship and identify potential outliers. The ranks of the absorbances at λ = 275 nm and the MOAH/MOSH ratios of various paraffin samples are listed in Tab. 3, the corresponding graph is shown in Fig. 1. As can be seen, a linear correlation between the ranks of the absorbances at λ = 275 nm and the MOAH/MOSH ratios was observed, except for the liquid paraffin samples 42 - 48 and 53. The $r_s$ values were calculated to be 0.503 for the whole dataset and 0.924

excluding the outlying liquid paraffin samples. The differences were investigated by evaluation of the corresponding spectroscopic results (Tab. 3). The UV absorbances of the outlying liquid paraffin samples were similar to those of the soft paraffin samples. In contrast, the MOAH/MOSH ratios of the liquid paraffins were much smaller compared to the soft paraffin samples.

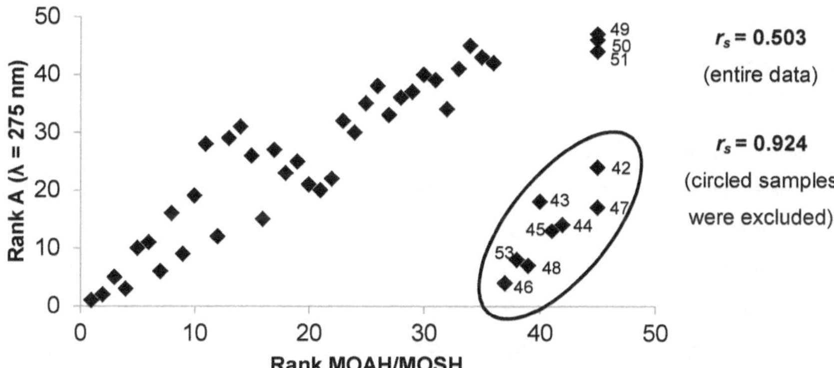


**Figure 1.** Rank correlation of UV absorbances (λ = 275 nm) and MOAH/MOSH ratios. The outlying liquid paraffin samples and their corresponding sample Nos. are shown encircled. $r_s$: Spearman's rank correlation coefficient.

Both UV and $^1$H NMR results showed that the synthetic liquid paraffins (49, 50, 51) contained comparably small amounts of aromatic compounds. The high UV absorbances of the outlying liquid paraffin samples 42 - 48 and 53 may be explained by the sample preparation (Tab. 1), where liquid paraffins are directly measured without preceding dilution. Hence, the eight liquid paraffin samples were withdrawn from further correlation models.

## 3.2 Linear regression of UV and NMR data

The results of the two measurement techniques for the determination of MAOH in paraffins were tested for a linear relationship, applying several correlation experiments. The absorbances obtained at λ = 275, 295 and > 300 nm were correlated with the MOAH/MOSH, PAH/MOSH and MAH/MOSH ratios of the paraffin samples, respectively, resulting in 9 correlation experiments (paraffin samples 42 - 48 and 53 were excluded). The correlation results were indicated by the $R^2$ values which are shown in Tab. 4.

**Table 4.** Correlation results of UV and NMR spectroscopic data of various paraffin samples, expressed as coefficients of determination $R^2$. The paraffin samples 42 - 48 and 53 were withdrawn from correlation experiments. A: absorbance; MAH: monocyclic aromatic hydrocarbons; MOAH: mineral oil hydrocarbons; PAH: polycyclic aromatic hydrocarbons.

|  | PAH/MOSH | MAH/MOSH | MOAH/MOSH |
|---|---|---|---|
| A ($\lambda$ = 275 nm) | 0.938 | 0.759 | 0.821 |
| A ($\lambda$ = 295 nm) | 0.977 | 0.626 | 0.726 |
| A ($\lambda$ > 300 nm) | 0.884 | 0.704 | 0.781 |

Overall, it was shown that the $^1$H NMR and UV spectroscopic data can be described by a linear model for the determination of MAOH in paraffins. The PAH/MOSH ratio showed the highest $R^2$ values for all wavelengths tested, whereas the MAH/MOSH ratio showed the lowest. The MOAH/MOSH ratio showed $R^2$ values in between. The PAH/MOSH ratios correlated well with the absorbances at $\lambda$ = 275 and 295 nm ($R^2$ = 0.938 and 0.977, respectively), slightly better than with the absorbances at $\lambda$ > 300 nm ($R^2$ = 0.884). Among the correlations of the MAH/MOSH ratios with the three wavelengths, $R^2$ was highest for $\lambda$ = 275 nm ($R^2$ = 0.759) and lowest for $\lambda$ = 295 nm ($R^2$ = 0.626). A similar trend was found for the MOAH/MOSH correlations.

## 3.3 Interpretation of correlation results

In the following, the interpretation of the correlation results was supported by the examination of how the amounts of PAH and MAH are presented by the UV/Vis and $^1$H NMR spectra.

## 3.3.1 Detection of MOAH in UV/Vis and $^1$H NMR spectroscopy

For the comparison of the UV and $^1$H NMR measurement results, it has to be considered that the degree of alkylation of the MOAH differently affects the evaluation of their amounts in the two methods. In UV/Vis spectroscopy, the number of alkyl substituents is expected to have a minor impact on the absorption bands of the MOAH. In contrast, in $^1$H NMR spectroscopy, the degree of substitution influences the number of the aromatic protons, which is proportional to the signal intensity.

In conclusion, the discrepancy between both methods increases with the degree of alkylation of the MOAH, resulting in lower $R^2$ values.

### 3.3.2 Evaluation of MOAH in the UV/Vis spectra of paraffins

As previously described, the UV test of the DAB 8 roughly assigns MOAH with one, two, and three or more aromatic rings to the wavelengths $\lambda$ = 275, 295 and > 300 nm, respectively. This was also indicated by the correlation results, where the MAH/MOSH and the PAH/MOSH ratios show the highest $R^2$ values for the correlations with the absorbances at $\lambda$ = 275 nm ($R^2$ = 0.759) and $\lambda$ = 295 nm (0.977), respectively (Tab. 4). However, in the UV/Vis spectrum, the PAH show absorbances over a large spectral range, which is due to the different number and connectivity of the aromatic rings and their degree of alkylation [11]. As a consequence, the absorbances of the MAH and PAH are likely to overlap at the measured wavelengths. In addition, as can be seen from the UV/Vis spectra of representative paraffin samples (Tab. 5), the absorbances at $\lambda$ = 275 and $\lambda$ > 300 nm were measured in slopes of the spectrum (at 295 nm, a small hump can be recognized), which leads to an increased fluctuation of the measured absorbances. Both circumstances may contribute to the comparatively low correlations of the MAH/MOSH ratios with the absorbances at $\lambda$ = 275 nm.

### 3.3.3 Evaluation of MOAH in the [1]H NMR spectra of paraffins

In the [1]H NMR spectra of the representative paraffin samples, the PAH could be distinguished more clearly from the MAH than in the UV/Vis spectra (Tab. 5), which facilitates the evaluation of the amount of MOAH. However, in contrast to the DAB 8, no distinction was made between PAH with two and more aromatic rings. It was shown that the amount of PAH is very low compared to the MAH, because the PAH are almost completely removed in several refining steps of paraffins for pharmaceutical use. Due to the more intense overlapping of the PAH and MAH, a corresponding evaluation was not feasible using the UV/Vis spectra.

**Table 5.** $^1$H NMR (recorded in CDCl$_3$) and UV/Vis spectra (recorded in isooctane) of the soft paraffin samples 9, 11 and 20 (low, medium and high amount of MOAH). Sample 20 was a non-hydrogenated paraffin intermediate. In the $^1$H NMR spectra, the regions of the MOAH protons are shown enlarged. MAH: monocyclic aromatic hydrocarbons; MOAH: mineral oil aromatic hydrocarbons; MOSH: mineral oil saturated hydrocarbons; PAH: polycyclic aromatic hydrocarbons.

**Sample 9**

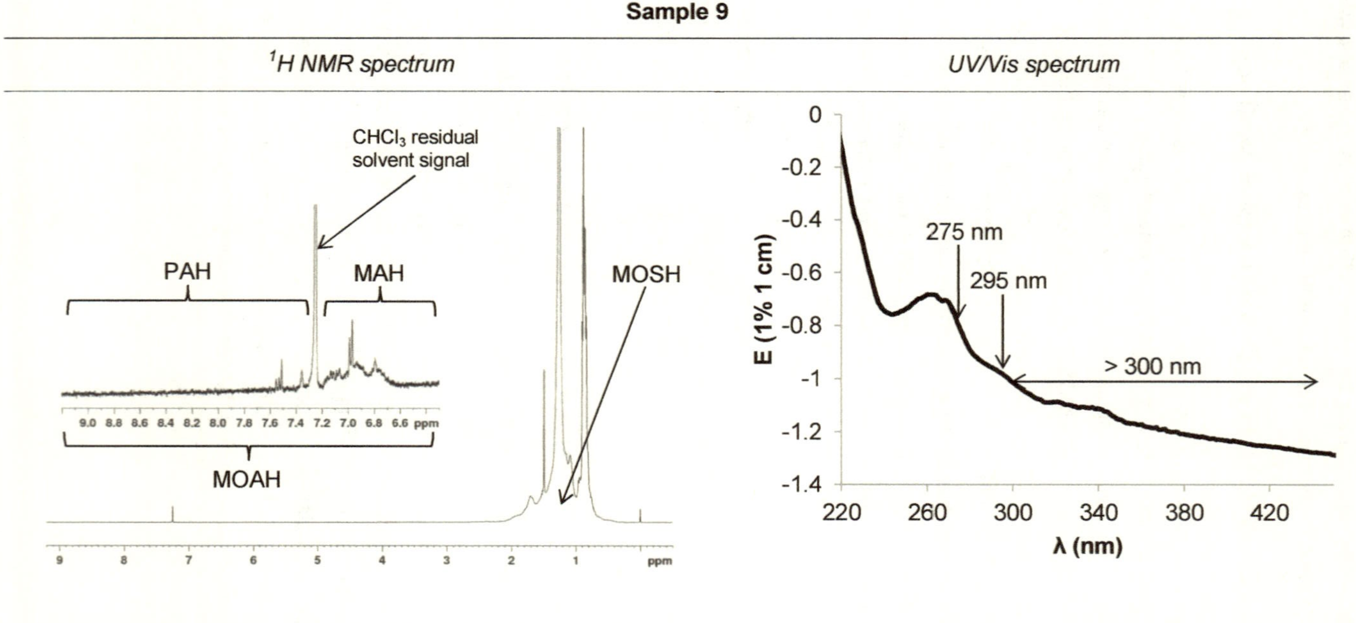

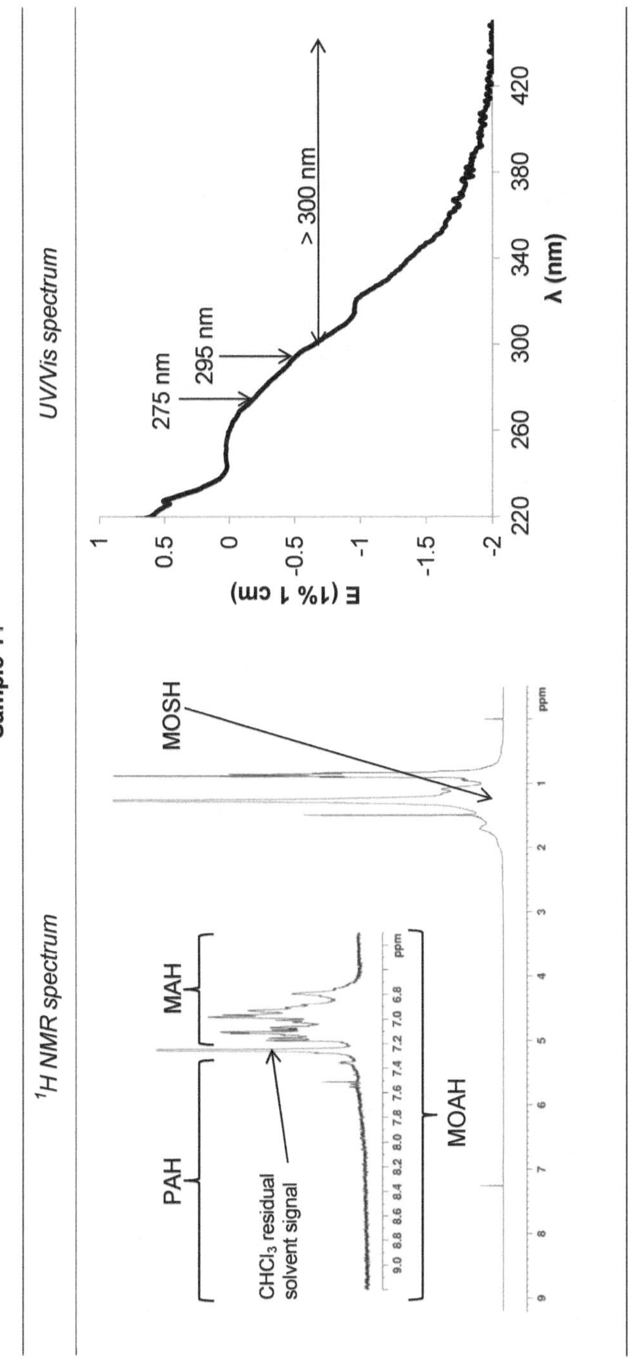
Sample 11
UV/Vis spectrum
$^1$H NMR spectrum
E (1% 1 cm)
λ (nm)
275 nm
295 nm
> 300 nm
MOSH
MAH
PAH
MOAH
CHCl₃ residual solvent signal
ppm

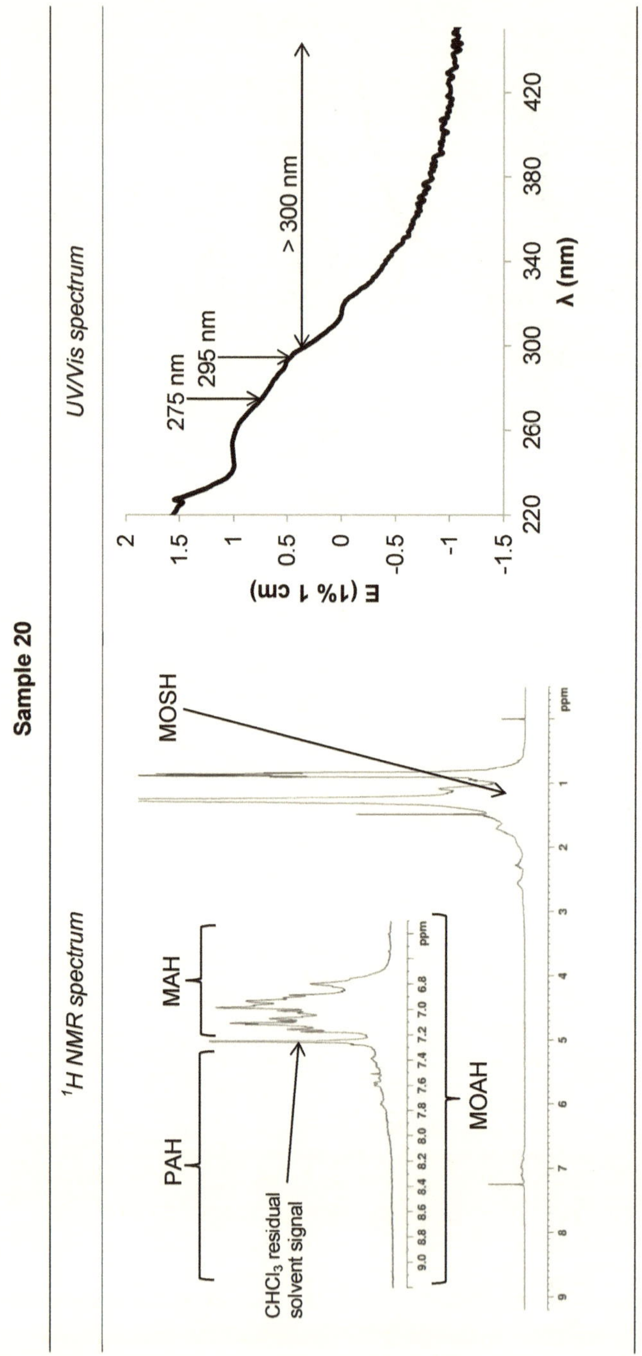
Sample 20
UV/Vis spectrum
275 nm
295 nm
> 300 nm
E (1% 1 cm)
2
1.5
1
0.5
0
-0.5
-1
-1.5
220
260
300
340
380
420
λ (nm)
$^1$H NMR spectrum
MOSH
MAH
PAH
MOAH
CHCl3 residual
solvent signal
9.0 8.8 8.6 8.4 8.2 8.0 7.8 7.6 7.4 7.2 7.0 6.8 ppm
ppm
1
2
3
4
5
6
7
8
9

# 4. Conclusion

For the evaluation of MOAH in paraffins, a large number of paraffin samples was analyzed by UV spectroscopy according to DAB 8 and compared to the $^1$H NMR spectroscopic results obtained in chapter 3.1.1. The absorbances at various wavelengths and the aromatic/aliphatic ratios from $^1$H NMR spectroscopic measurements showed an approximately linear relationship. However, the correlation results should be carefully used for assigning the tested wavelengths to a spectral region within the $^1$H NMR spectrum, as they are affected by the varying degree of alkylation and overlapping resonances/absorbances of the MOAH.

# 5. References

[1] Hochraffinierte Mineralöle in Kosmetika: Gesundheitliche Risiken sind nach derzeitigem Kenntnisstand nicht zu erwarten. Aktualisierte Stellungnahme Nr. 008/2018 des BfR, 27. Februar 2018.

[2] Kommentar zum Europäischen Arzneibuch, Monographie 8.0/1799 – Weißes Vaselin. 52. Aktualisierungslieferung, Wissenschaftliche Verlagsgesellschaft Stuttgart, Stuttgart, 2015.

[3] A. Dooms-Goossens, H. Degreef, Contact allergy to petrolatums (I). Sensitizing capacity of different brands of yellow and white petrolatums. Contact Dermatitis 1983, 9, 175-185.

[4] A. Dooms-Goossens, H. Degreef, Contact allergy to petrolatums (II). Attempts to identify the nature of the allergens. Contact Dermatitis 1983, 9, 247-256.

[5] H. Böhme, W. Hühnermann, Probleme des Arzneibuches. Zur Untersuchung der Mineralölprodukte im Deutschen Arzneibuch, 7. Ausgabe. Arch. Pharm. 1966, 299, 368-380.

[6] S.A. Schou, I. Bendix-Nielsen, Untersuchungen über die Reinheit der Paraffinöle. Arch. Pharm. 1934, 272, 761-169.

[7] Deutsches Arzneibuch, Monographie Weisses Vaselin. 8. Ausgabe (DAB 8) - Amtliche Ausgabe, Govi-Verlag GmbH, Frankfurt, Deutscher Apotheker-Verlag, Stuttgart, 1978.

[8] Deutsches Arzneibuch, Monographie Dickflüssiges Paraffin. 8. Ausgabe (DAB 8) - Amtliche Ausgabe, Govi-Verlag GmbH, Frankfurt, Deutscher Apotheker-Verlag, Stuttgart, 1978.

[9] Deutsches Arzneibuch, Monographie Dünnflüssiges Paraffin. 8. Ausgabe (DAB 8) - Amtliche Ausgabe, Govi-Verlag GmbH, Frankfurt, Deutscher Apotheker-Verlag, Stuttgart, 1978.

[10] Deutsches Arzneibuch, Monographie Hartparaffin. 8. Ausgabe (DAB 8) - Amtliche Ausgabe, Govi-Verlag GmbH, Frankfurt, Deutscher Apotheker-Verlag, Stuttgart, 1978.

[11] E. Pretsch, P. Bühlmann, M. Badertscher, Spektroskopische Daten zur Strukturaufklärung organischer Verbindungen. 5. Auflage, Springer, Berlin, Heidelberg, 2010.

[12] Ph.Eur. EDQM, Strasbourg, France. Monograph No. 1799 – Paraffin, White Soft. European Pharmacopoeia Online 10.4, 2020.

[13] DAB 9 Kommentar, Deutsches Arzneibuch, 9. Ausgabe 1986 mit wissenschaftlichen Erläuterungen. Monographie Weißes Vaselin. Wissenschaftliche Verlagsgesellschaft Stuttgart, Stuttgart, 1988.

[14] S. Weber, K. Schrag, G. Mildau, T. Kuballa, S.G. Walch, D.W. Lachenmeier, Analytical Methods for the Determination of Mineral Oil Saturated Hydrocarbons (MOSH) and Mineral Oil Aromatic Hydrocarbons (MOAH) – A Short Review. Anal. Chem. Insights 2018, 13, 1-16.

[15] K. Siebertz, D. van Bebber, T. Hochkirchen, Statistische Versuchsplanung: Design of Experiments (DoE). 2. Auflage, Springer Vieweg, Berlin, Heidelberg, 2017.

[16] F. Rohlf, R.R. Sokal, Statistical Tables. Freeman and Co., San Francisco, 1969.

[17] H. Böhme, K. Hartke, DAB 8 Kommentar, Deutsches Arzneibuch, 8. Ausgabe 1978, Monographie Dickflüssiges Paraffin. Wissenschaftliche Verlagsgesellschaft Stuttgart, Stuttgart, Govi-Verlag GmbH, Frankfurt, 1981.

[18] Ph.Eur. EDQM, Strasbourg, France. Chapter 2.2.25 – Absorption Spectrophotometry, Ultraviolet and Visible. European Pharmacopoeia Online 10.4, 2020.

# 3.1.4 Characterization of paraffins by means of principal component analysis

## 1. Introduction

NMR spectra provide a high amount of information. However, the interpretation of spectra with highly overlapping resonances is difficult, which applies e.g. to multi-component mixtures. For extracting the hidden information out of such large data sets, chemometric (multivariate) techniques such as the principal component analysis (PCA) can be applied [1-3]. PCA is an unsupervised, explorative chemometric tool, which is used to identify clusters and patterns within the dataset. This is accomplished by decomposing the spectral information into the principal components (PCs) or the so-called latent variables to visualize the main variation in the data [4].

In the present work, a first approach to PCA of the $^1$H NMR spectra of various paraffin samples for pharmaceutical use (see chapter 3.1.1) was performed in order to examine the extent to which a discrimination of paraffins is possible, and which variables are responsible for the differentiation or the formation of the groups within the paraffin samples.

## 2. Experimental section

### 2.1 Materials and methods

### 2.1.1 Paraffin samples and $^1$H NMR data

The $^1$H NMR spectra of 54 paraffins for pharmaceutical and technical use from 9 manufacturers, including 34 soft, 12 liquid (including 3 synthetic paraffins) and 5 solid paraffins (including 3 synthetic waxes) and 3 refining intermediates, were subjected to PCA. A detailed overview of the paraffin samples and the corresponding $^1$H NMR data is given in chapter 3.1.1.

### 2.1.2 Principal component analysis

The principles and mathematical fundamentals of PCA will not be discussed in detail, but are comprehensively described in the literature, e.g. in [4-7]. The score matrix T was composed of n rows (samples) and p columns (factors/PCs), the loading matrix $P^T$ of p rows (factors) and m columns (variables, i.e. $^1H$ NMR spectral data points as a function of chemical shift). Interpretation of scores and loadings was performed in order to identify sample groupings, as well as the variables contributing to it.

Prior to PCA, the NMR spectra were transformed into buckets of a width of 0.05 ppm using Amix (Bruker Biospin GmbH, Rheinstetten, Germany). The bucketing procedure is performed in order to achieve data reduction by grouping spectral regions into a bucket of a predefined width, which covers the sum of intensities of the respective spectral region. The buckets of the $^1H$ NMR spectra were scaled to unit variance.

PCA was performed using the Unscrambler X version 11.0 (Camo Software AS, Oslo, Norway). The PCA models were established on the mean centered data applying the singular value decomposition algorithm and a cross validation procedure. The $^1H$ NMR data was subjected to PCA using five PCs. Due to the highly varying signal intensities within a spectrum, each spectral region of interest was evaluated independently using PCA.

## 3. Results and discussion

### 3.1 $^1H$ NMR spectra of paraffins

Paraffins are multi-component mixtures, consisting of mineral oil hydrocarbons (MOH) with different chain lengths and branching [8]. Generally, the MOH are divided into the mineral oil saturated hydrocarbons (MOSH) and the mineral oil aromatic hydrocarbons (MOAH). The latter comprise compounds with one (monocyclic aromatic hydrocarbons, MAH) and two or more aromatic rings (polycyclic aromatic hydrocarbons). Paraffins for pharmaceutical use are dominated by the MOSH fraction, whereas the MOAH occur in small amounts of a few percent (depending on the extent of refining).

A typical $^1H$ NMR spectrum of a representative soft paraffin sample is shown in Fig. 1. The most intense integral between $\delta = 0.16$ and 4.0 ppm is referred to the MOSH protons. Among the MOSH, a differentiation is possible between the alkane and benzylic $CH_2$ and $CH_3$ groups, respectively. The MOAH signals were integrated from $\delta$ = 6.5 - 9.1 ppm ($CHCl_3$ signal was excluded, $\delta$ = 7.22 - 7.3 ppm), which were roughly assigned to the MAH ($\delta$ = 6.5 - 7.22 ppm) and the PAH ($\delta$ = 7.3 - 9.1 ppm).

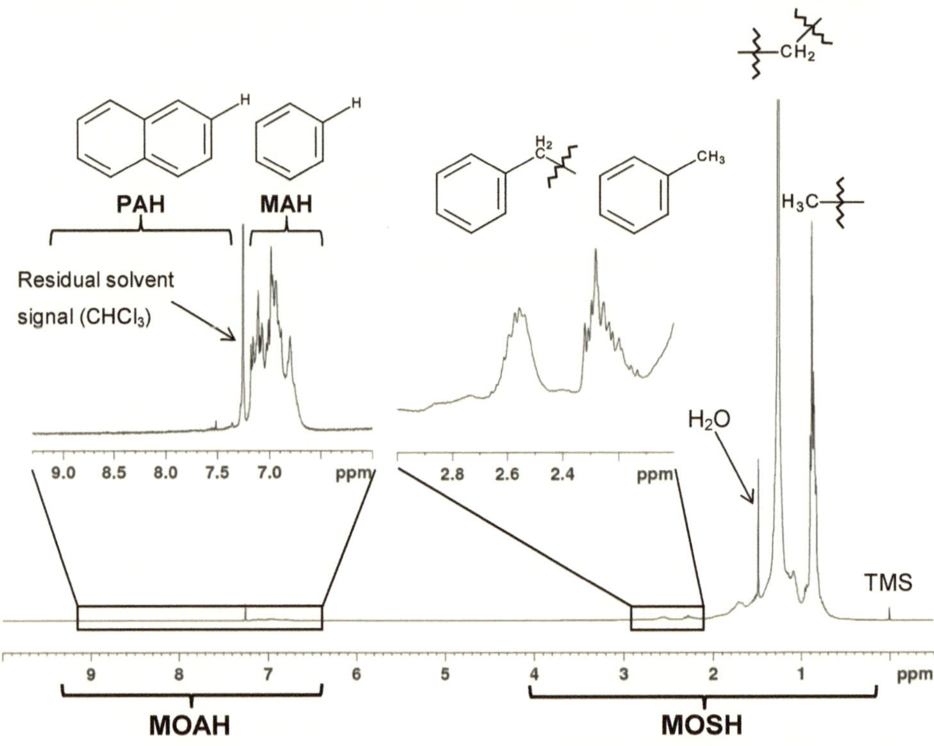


**Figure 1.** Representative $^1$H NMR spectrum of soft paraffin sample D (recorded in $CDCl_3$). A selection of MOH structures was assigned to the spectral regions. MAH, monocyclic aromatic hydrocarbons; MOAH, mineral oil aromatic hydrocarbons; MOSH, mineral oil saturated hydrocarbons; PAH, polycyclic aromatic hydrocarbons; TMS, tetramethylsilane (reference standard).

## 3.2 PCA of $^1$H NMR spectroscopic data

First, to get an overview of the data, a PCA model was established including all paraffin samples and the spectral regions of the MOSH and MOAH. The first two principal components explained 98% of the total variance. As can be seen in the score plot of PC-1 versus PC-2, a separation into three groups along PC-1 (81% variance), liquid, soft and solid paraffins, could be observed (Fig. 2). PC-2 (17% variance) separated natural and synthetic liquid paraffin samples. The soft paraffin samples were located around the center of the score plot, which means that those samples are not sufficiently described by the PCA model.

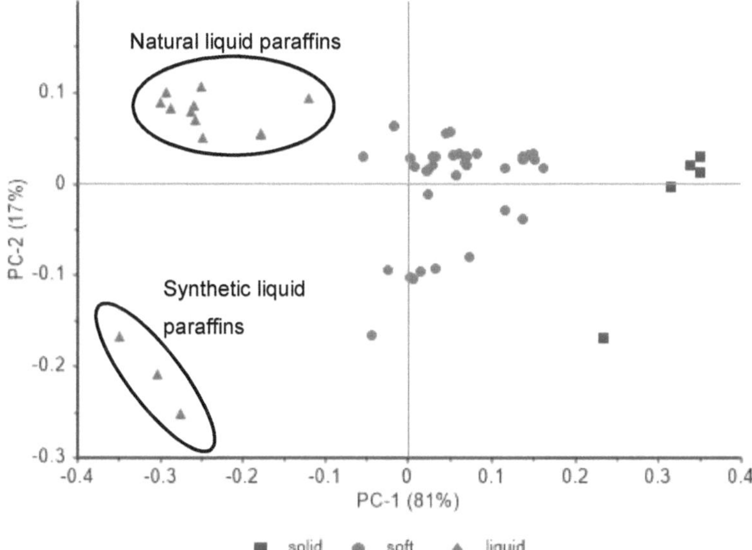


**Figure 2.** Score plot of PC-1 vs. PC-2. Triangles, liquid paraffins; circles, soft paraffins; squares, solid paraffins. Groupings within the liquid paraffins are encircled.

In order to determine the $^1$H NMR spectral regions (chemical shifts) responsible for the groupings, the corresponding loading plots were evaluated (Fig. 3). The loadings of PC-1 indicate the maximum variance within the $^1$H NMR spectra is located in the MOSH region (aliphatic $CH_2$ and $CH_3$ groups, Fig. 3). This is comprehensible because the MOSH are the predominant species in paraffins, and the structural composition of the MOSH is characteristic for liquid, solid and soft paraffins [8-10]. For example, liquid paraffins mainly contain iso- and cyclic MOH of low chain lengths, whereas solid paraffins are composed of *n*-alkanes.

The differentiation between natural and synthetic liquid paraffins along PC-2 may be also due to their MOH composition. The loadings of PC-2 (Fig. 4) ascribe the most variance to the aliphatic $CH_2$ groups of the MOH, which may be explained by the manufacturing process of the synthetic paraffins: they are commonly produced by the Fischer-Tropsch process, which almost exclusively results in mixtures of straight-chain alkanes with a sharp carbon distribution [11]. In contrast, the natural liquid paraffins are mainly composed of iso- and cyclic alkanes. A distinction between natural and synthetic solid paraffins could not be made, which may be due to the small structural differences of the MOH in those paraffins.

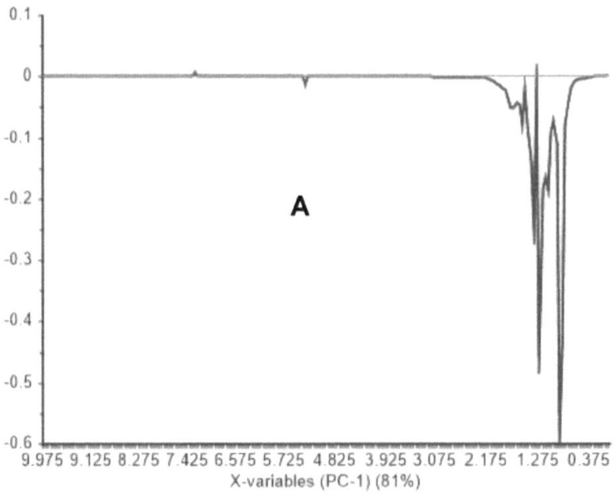


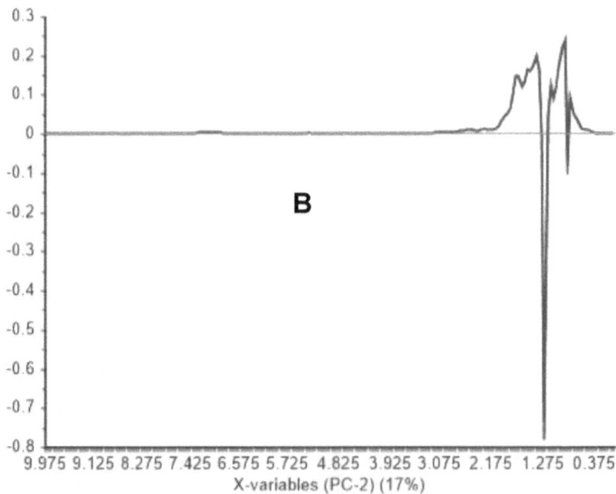


**Figure 3.** Loading plots of PC-1 and PC-2. (A) PC-1 (81% total variance); the main variance is ascribed to the alkane $CH_2$ and $CH_3$ groups of the MOSH. (B) PC-2 (17% total variance); The main variance of both PCs is due to the MOSH protons of the paraffins.

Groupings according to other characteristics such as the MOAH/MOSH ratio, solubility (determined in chapter 3.1.1), type, or manufacturer of the paraffin samples were not observed with this PCA model. Additional models built from reduced sample matrices, including e.g. samples from one manufacturer or one paraffin type, also did not result in satisfactory discrimination of the samples: Fig. 4 shows the score plot of PC-1 versus PC-2 of soft and solid paraffin samples, assigned to the solubility in $CDCl_3$ at 313 K (mg/mL). Fig. 5 depicts the score plot of PC-1 versus PC-2 of the soft paraffin samples intended for pharmaceutical use, assigned to various manufacturers. Further models were established by subjecting the MOAH regions to PCA, because small variations in the spectral data of the paraffins may not be distinguished due to the comparatively huge amount of the MOSH. However, no sample groupings could be observed using those models.

The projection of other PCs (apart from PC-1 versus PC-2) against each other did not result in improved sample separation in neither PCA model.

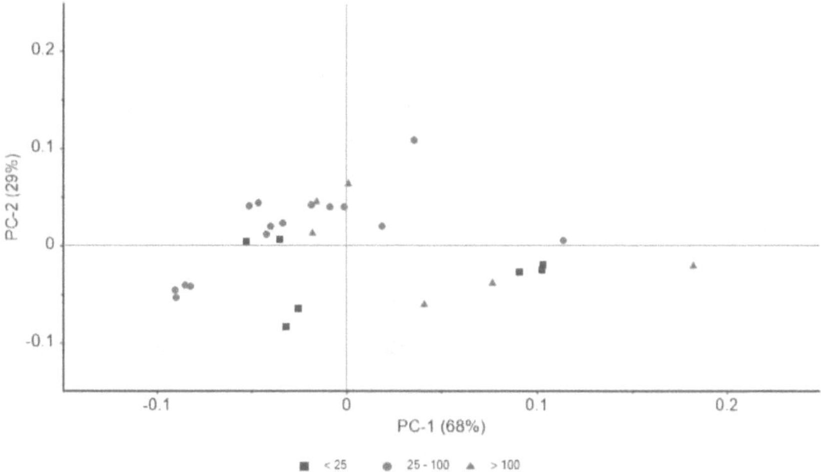


**Figure 4.** Score plot of PC-1 vs. PC-2. Data input for modelling: soft and solid paraffins, assigned to their solubilty in $CDCl_3$ at 313 K. < 25 mg/mL (squares), 25 - 100 mg/mL (circles), > 100 mg/mL (triangles).

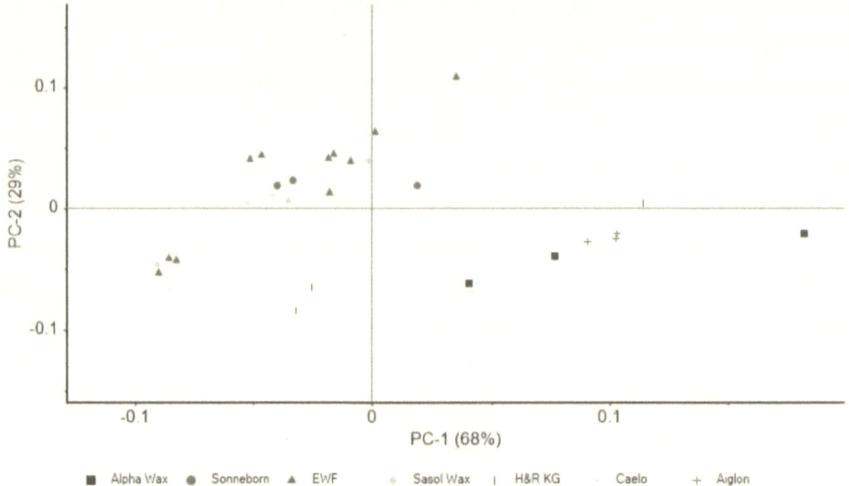

**Figure 5.** Score plot of PC-1 vs. PC-2. Data input for modelling: soft paraffins for pharmacutical use, assigned to various manufacturers.

## 4. Conclusion

In this project, first approaches were made to distinguish between various paraffin samples measured by $^1$H NMR spectroscopy using PCA. Groupings were mainly due to the variances of the MOSH. A differentiation could be made between solid, liquid and soft paraffins on the one hand, and between natural and synthetic liquid paraffins on the other hand. Sample groupings according to other characteristics, such as solubility or manufacturers, could not be observed. PCA models including only the spectral regions of the MOAH were found to be inadequate to resolve the paraffin samples.

The data set used for PCA contains many different paraffin samples, so it would be interesting to use them also for classification procedures (e.g. soft independent modelling of class analogy, SIMCA) and regression methods (e.g. principal component regression, PCR), which is, however, not part of this work. Moreover, the model can be complemented with additional paraffin samples to increase the reliability of the results.

## 5. References

[1] Y.B. Monakhova, U. Holzgrabe, B.W.K. Diehl, Current role and future perspective of multivariate (chemometric) methods in NMR spectroscopic analysis of pharmaceutical products. J. Pharm. Biomed. Anal. 2018, 147, 580-589.

[2] H. Winning, F.H. Larsen, R. Bro, S.B. Engelsen, Quantitative analysis of NMR spectra with chemometrics. J. Magn. Reson. 2008, 190, 26-32.

[3] J.S. McKenzie, J.A. Donarski, J.C. Wilson, A.J. Charlton, Analysis of complex mixtures using high-resolution nuclear magnetic resonance spectroscopy and chemometrics. Progr. Nucl. Magn. Reson. Spectrosc. 2011, 59, 336-359.

[4] EDQM, Strasbourg, France. Chapter 5.21 – Chemometric Methods Applied To Analytical Data. European Pharmacopoeia Online 10.4, 2020.

[5] S. Wold, K. Esbensen, P. Geladi, Principal component analysis. Chemom. Intell. Lab. Syst. 1987, 2, 37-52.

[6] H. Abdi, L.J. Williams, Principal component analysis. Wiley Interdisc. Rev.: Comput. Stat. 2010, 2, 433-459.

[7] R. Stoyanova, T.R. Brown, NMR spectral quantitation by principal component analysis. NMR Biomed. 2001, 14, 271-277.

[8] Kommentar zum Europäischen Arzneibuch, Monographie 8.0/1799 – Weißes Vaselin. 52. Aktualisierungslieferung, Wissenschaftliche Verlagsgesellschaft Stuttgart, Stuttgart, 2015.

[9] Kommentar zum Europäischen Arzneibuch, Monographie 5.0/0239 – Dickflüssiges Paraffin. 52. Aktualisierungslieferung, Wissenschaftliche Verlagsgesellschaft Stuttgart, Stuttgart, 2015.

[10] Kommentar zum Europäischen Arzneibuch, Monographie 6.0/1034 – Hartparaffin. 52. Aktualisierungslieferung, Wissenschaftliche Verlagsgesellschaft Stuttgart, Stuttgart, 2015.

[11] D. Sothmann, K. Südkamp, Aufreinigung von Mineralöl für den Einsatz in kosmetischen Mitteln und Arzneimitteln, in: Mineralöl im Fokus des

gesundheitlichen Verbraucherschutzes, BfR-Forum 7./8. Dezember 2017, Berlin. Available from: https://www.bfr.bund.de/de/veranstaltung/mineraloel_im_fokus_des_gesundheitlichen_verbraucherschutzes-203107.html. Accessed May 10th 2021.

## 3.2 Impurity profiling of L-ascorbic acid 2-phosphate magnesium using NMR spectroscopy [*]

## 1. Introduction

L-Ascorbic acid (AsA, Fig. 1), also known as vitamin C, plays an important role in many biochemical processes. In the human body, it acts as an antioxidant, preventing the formation of reactive oxidative species (ROS) and free radicals [1,2]. It is involved in the production of collagen, adrenocorticosteroids and several neurotransmitters such as serotonin and norepinephrine.

However, AsA is not suitable for long term studies in cell media due to its rapid decomposition in aqueous environment, exposure to oxygen, heat, and light [1,3]. The high reducing potential and instability of AsA is ascribed to the endiol group at C-2 and C-3. The phosphorylation of C-2 leads to L-ascorbic acid 2-phosphate (A2P), which is found to be stable under the abovementioned conditions *in vitro*, but is metabolized into AsA by alkaline phosphatases *in vivo* [4]. L-ascorbic acid 2-phosphate magnesium (A2PMg, Fig. 2) has an improved stability and can be used under common culture media conditions for cell and tissue regenerating therapies [3,5,6].

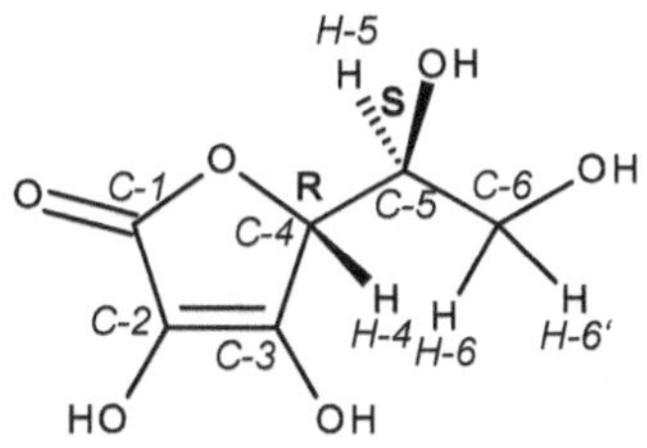

**Figure 1.** Structure of AsA.

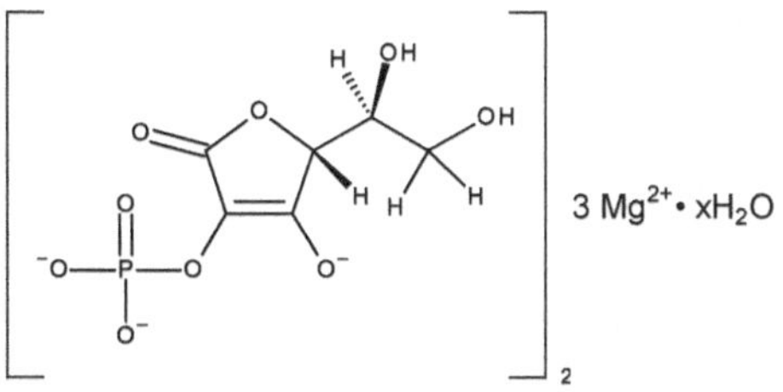

**Figure 2.** Structure of A2PMg.

---

[*] Parts of the results presented in this chapter have been published in [18], which is reprinted in the appendix (section 7.5) for supporting information. The paper is not treated as part of this book and not listed in "Documentation of Authorship" (section 7.2), because the author of the book contributed to the paper to only about 10%. The present chapter gives more detailed information about the impurity profiling of A2PMg by NMR spectroscopy and provides additional research findings.

Many manufacturing processes of AsA phosphate esters and salts thereof have been reported [7-15]. In general, the reactions were carried out in an aqueous solution of a tertiary amine, e.g. pyridine, at pH > 8 and low temperatures (-10 - 10 °C) [10,12]. Using phosphorus oxyhalides such as $POCl_3$, unprotected AsA was directly phosphorylated, or the 5- and 6-OH groups of AsA were protected before phosphorylation. Process variations included adjustments of reaction temperature, solvents, amount or ratio of reagents.

Apart from unreacted starting materials, several by-products can occur. Phosphorylation of the hydroxyl groups at C-2, C-3, C-5 and/or C-6 results in compound mixtures, including 2-pyrophosphates, bis(L-ascorbic acid)2,2'-phosphate, bis(L-ascorbic acid)2,3'-phosphate and bis(L-ascorbic acid)3,3'-phosphate [9,14]. Besides, if methanol was used as reaction solvent, L-ascorbic methylphosphates were formed [15].

Furthermore, impurities resulting from decomposition of AsA and its phosphorylated derivatives have to be considered. The hydrolysis of A2PMg phosphate esters has been thoroughly investigated, which mainly results in the formation of AsA by a P-O bond cleavage [9,16]. In aqueous solution, AsA is oxidized to dehydro ascorbic acid, which is further hydrolyzed to 2,3-diketogulonic acid, oxalic acid and threonic acid [1,17]. Furthermore, AsA derivatives, which are phosphorylated on the C-3 position, are converted into the more stable A2P and AsA by acid catalyzed hydrolysis and concurrent migration of the 3-phosphate group [9].

Up to now, little has been reported on the pharmaceutical quality control of the A2PMg substance. Xu et al. developed a hydrophilic interaction liquid chromatography (HILIC) method for the purity evaluation of crude A2PMg purchased from different suppliers [18]. Using HPLC with high resolution MS and MS/MS detection, three related impurities (Imps) with an m/z of 283 could be detected, which were assumed to be variously ethylated derivatives of the A2PMg substance (Fig. 3). Although ethylated by-products have not been reported yet, their formation is conceivable, because ethanol is used as a recrystallization agent in the preparation of A2PMg.

The aim of this study was to support the MS data using NMR spectroscopy, focusing on structural elucidation of the A2PMg impurities. For this purpose, the impurity fractions collected from preparative liquid chromatography (LC) of A2PMg were analyzed.

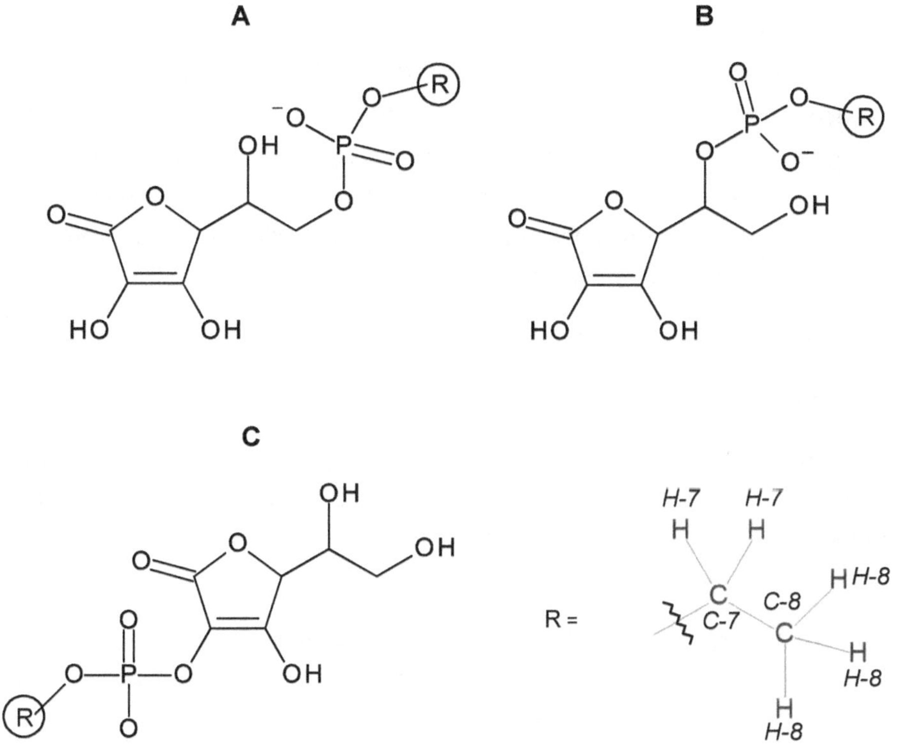

**Figure 3.** A2PMg impurities found by Xu et al. [18]. (A) Impurity 1; (B) impurity 2; (C) impurity 3.

## 2. Experimental section

### 2.1 Chemicals and materials

Deuteriumoxide ($D_2O \geq 99.96$ atom % D) was purchased from Sigma-Aldrich Chemie GmbH (Steinheim, Germany) and 3-(trimethylsilyl)propionic-2,2,3,3-$d_4$ acid sodium salt (TSP $\geq$ 98%) from Alfa Aesar (Kandel, Germany). The A2PMg sample was obtained from Discovery fine chemicals (product code S22-24/25, lot#75380; Wimborne, UK). The isolated fractions from preparative LC were provided by the Drug Quality and Registration (DruQuaR) Group, Faculty of Pharmaceutical Sciences, Ghent University, Ghent, Belgium. pH-indicator strips were purchased from Merck KGaA (Darmstadt, Germany).

### 2.2 Apparatus and equipment

For the NMR measurements, the following instruments were used.

Bruker Avance III HD 600 MHz spectrometer with cryoplatform, equipped with a DCH $^{13}C/^1H$ cryoprobe with z gradient and ATM, a SampleXpress automatic sample changer, and a BCU1 variable temperature precooling unit. The temperature during measurements was 295 K.

Bruker Avance III HD 600 MHz Ascend spectrometer was equipped with a BBFO probe with z gradient and ATM, a BACS 120 automatic sample changer, and a BCU2 variable temperature precooling unit, operating at 295 K.

The $^1H$ NMR spectra were recorded using the Bruker standard zg30 pulse sequence (pulse angle 30°). Other acquisition parameters are described in the text. For spectra processing and analysis, the Bruker TopSpin 4.0.8 software was used. $^1H$ and $^{13}C$ NMR spectra were referenced with respect to the TSP signal at $\delta = 0$ ppm.

### 2.3 Sample preparation for NMR measurements

About 15 mg of the A2PMg substance or 5 mg of the isolated LC fraction were dissolved in 700 µL or 5000 µL $D_2O$ (containing 0.03 mg/mL TSP), respectively. The apparent pH values of the resulting solutions were measured to be $\sim$ 7 for the crude A2PMg substance and $\sim$ 1 for the isolated fractions, using pH-indicator strips. To correct for $D_2O$ solutions, it is defined $pH_D = pH_{apparent} + 0.4$ [19], so the true $pH_D$

values are expected to be slightly higher. 650 µL of the respective mixture were transferred into a 5 mm NMR tube for measurement.

## 3. Results and discussion

### 3.1 NMR measurements of crude A2PMg

Fig. 4 shows the [1]H NMR spectrum of A2PMg. The signal assignment of H-4 (1H, $\delta$ = 4.59 ppm, d), H-5 (1H, $\delta$ = 4.10 ppm, m) and H-6/H-6' (2H, $\delta$ = 3.76, m) was based on data of A2P reported in [9,20]. The splitting patterns are due to the second order ABMX spin system: A (H-6), B (H-6'), M (H-5), X (H-4) [21].

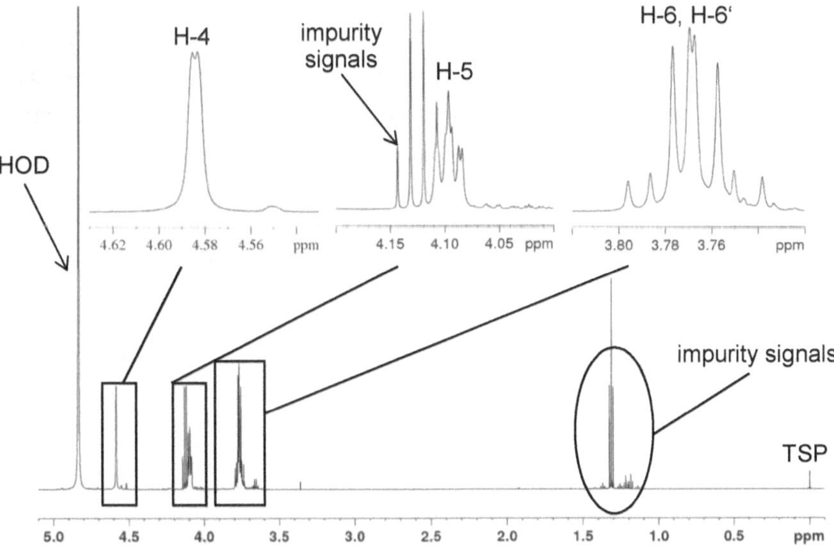


**Figure 4.** [1]H NMR spectrum of A2PMg in $D_2O$ (pH 7). 600 MHz, BBFO probe, number of scans (NS): 1024, size of FID: 147456. Signals of H-4 (1H, $\delta$ = 4.59 ppm), H-5 (1H, $\delta$ = 4.10 ppm), H-6/H-6' (2H, $\delta$ = 3.76 ppm) and impurity signals ($\delta$ = 4.12 ppm) are shown enlarged. TSP: 3-(trimethylsilyl)propionic-2,2,3,3-$d_4$ acid sodium salt.

Additional triplets (3H methyl protons, H-8, Fig. 5A) and quartets (2H methylene protons, H-7, Fig. 5B-D) from $\delta$ = 1.1 - 1.5 ppm and $\delta$ = 3.65 - 4.71 ppm, respectively ($^3J_{H7,H8}$ = 7.1 Hz), could be observed. Using $^{13}$C, COSY, HSQC and HMBC experiments, seven pairs of triplets and quartets of ethyl groups of several impurities could be assigned to impurites *a - g* (Fig. 5 and 6). Among them, the residual solvent ethanol (methyl 3H, $\delta$ = 1.18 ppm; methylene 2H, $\delta$ = 3.65 ppm) could be identified by spiking to the sample solution. In the $^{13}$C NMR spectrum of A2PMg, the C-7 and C-8 signals of the ethylated impurities were found from $\delta$ = 14 - 17 ppm and $\delta$ = 57 - 69 ppm, respectively (Fig. 6A,B).

The methyl and methylene signals of the ethyl groups show large differences in their chemical shifts ($\delta$ = 1.14 - 1.46 ppm and 3.65 - 4.71 ppm, respectively), indicating that the ethyl group is attached to different positions of the AsA skeleton in those impurities. The methylene protons of impurities *c* and *d* resonate at about $\delta$ = 4.05 and 4.11 ppm, respectively, which may indicate an ethylated phosphate ester such as $CH_3CH_2$-$PO_4$-AsA [22]. The chemical shifts of the methylene signals of impurities *e* ($\delta$ = 3.66 ppm), *f* ($\delta$ = 3.65 ppm) and *g* ($\delta$ = 3.70 ppm) are indicative for ethyl ethers attached to the AsA molecule similar to $CH_3CH_2$-O-AsA. The methylene signals of impurity *b* are substantially downfield shifted to $\delta$ = 4.71 ppm, indicating the ethyl group is not attached to the AsA skeleton, but to moieties with strong electron-withdrawing effects such as carboxylic acids, esters, or halogenes.

**A**

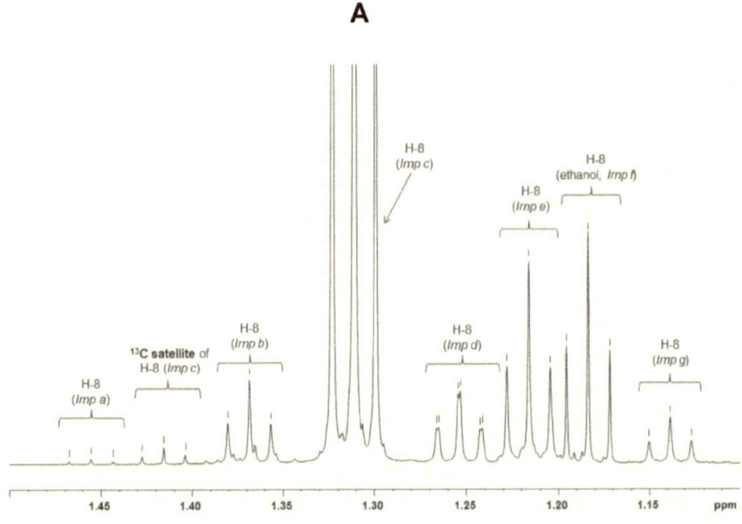

# Impurity profiling of L-ascorbic acid 2-phosphate magnesium using NMR spectroscopy

**B**

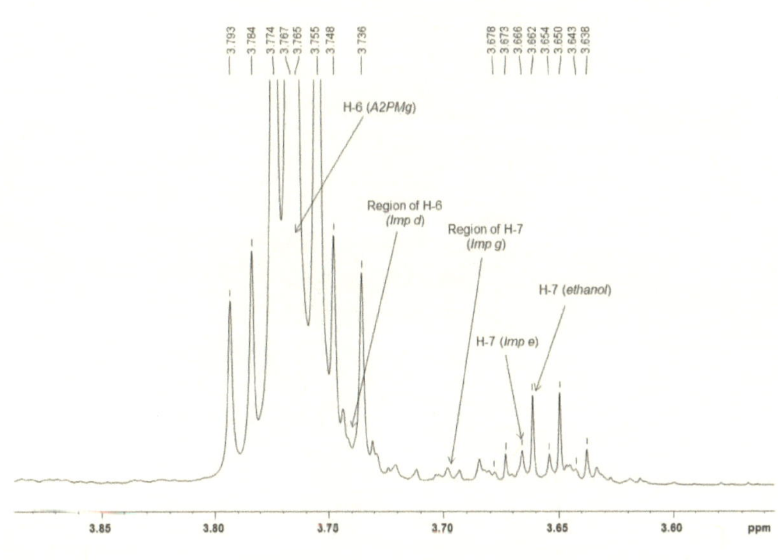


**C**

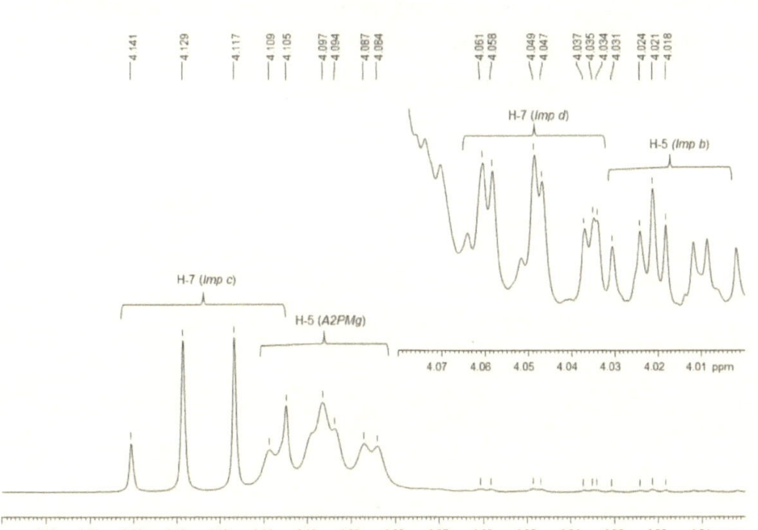

**D**

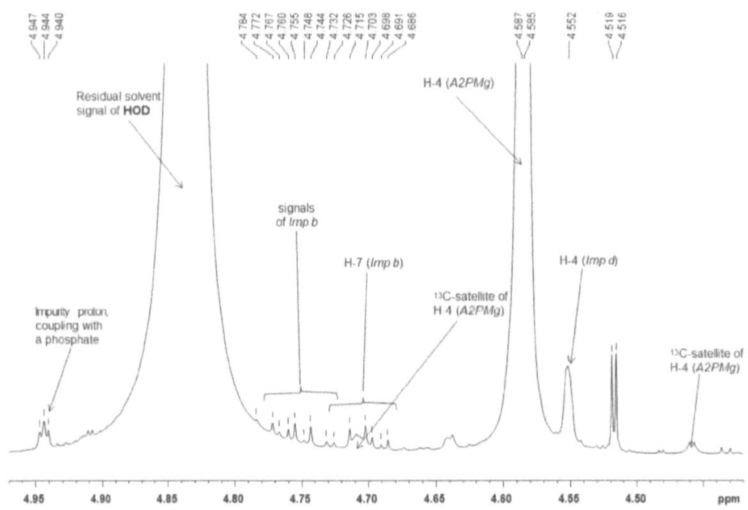


**Figure 5.** Signal assignments in expanded parts of the $^1$H NMR spectrum of A2PMg in D$_2$O (pH 7). 600 MHz, BBFO probe, NS: 1024, size of FID: 147456. (A) spectral region δ = 1.1 - 1.5 ppm, showing the H-8 signals of several ethylated impurities a - g; (B) spectral region δ = 3.55 - 3.9 ppm; (C) spectral region δ = 3.9 - 4.2 ppm; (D) spectral region δ = 4.45 - 4.98 ppm.

# Impurity profiling of L-ascorbic acid 2-phosphate magnesium using NMR spectroscopy

## A

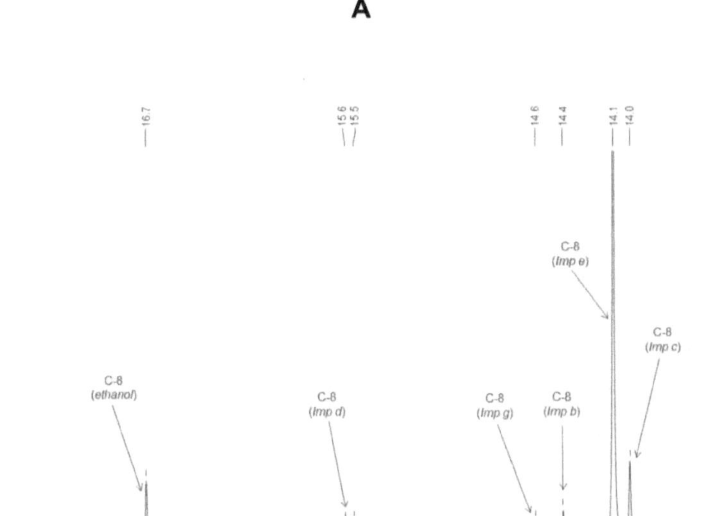


## B

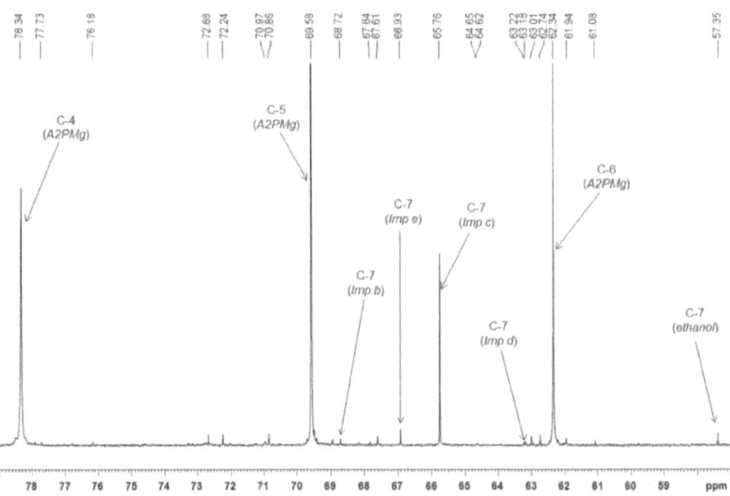

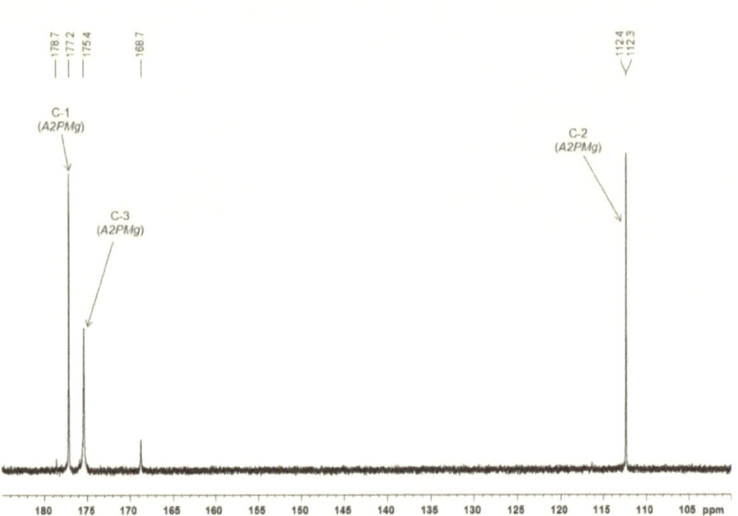

**Figure 6.** Signal assignments in expanded parts of the $^{13}$C NMR spectrum of A2PMg in $D_2O$ (pH 7). 600 MHz, BBFO probe, NS: 1024, size of FID: 147456. (A) spectral region $\delta$ = 13 - 18 ppm, (B) spectral region $\delta$ = 57 - 79 ppm; (C) spectral region $\delta$ = 100 - 185 ppm.

Identification of the positions and potential substituents of phosphate esters was performed by evaluation of the $^{31}$P-$^{1}$H couplings. The $^{5}J_{P-H}$ long-range coupling of the phosphorus ($\delta$ = 1.096 ppm) to H-4 of A2PMg could be observed ($^{5}J_{H,P}$ ~ 0.8 Hz), but not to the H-5 or H-6 protons (Fig. 7). Contrary to reports in the literature [9], no splitting of the $^{31}$P signal could be detected. Among the ethylated impurities *a - g*, only the protons of impurity *d* showed several cross peaks: H-4 ($\delta$ = 4.55 ppm, $^{5}J_{H,P}$ ~ 0.8 Hz), H-7 ($\delta$ = 4.05 ppm, $^{3}J_{H,P}$ ~ 7.1 Hz) and H-8 ($\delta$ = 1.25 ppm, $^{4}J_{H,P}$ ~ 0.8 Hz) couple to the phosphorus at $\delta$ = -2.265 ppm, indicating an ethyl phosphate ester on C-2 of A2PMg, which strongly suggests the structure of impurity 3 (Fig. 3C) [22]. Other detected $^{31}$P-$^{1}$H couplings indicate several phosphorylated compounds which were most likely formed during synthesis. However, the structure could not be elucidated. An overview of the spectroscopic data is given in Tab. 1.

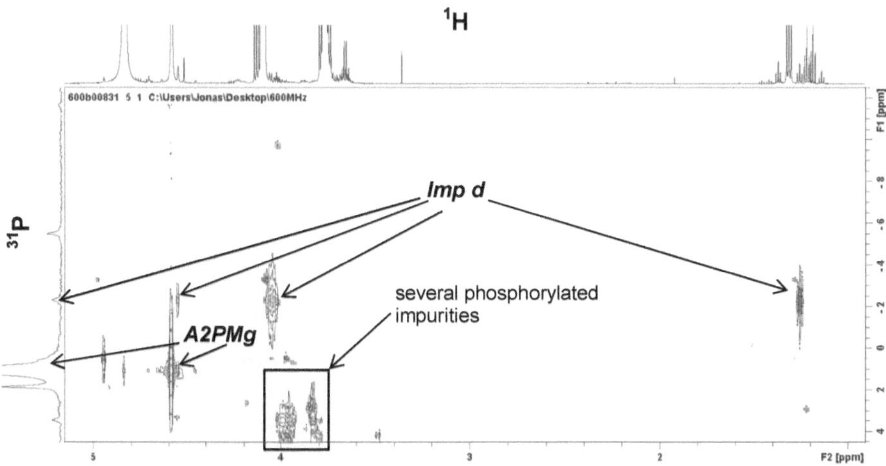



**Figure 7.** H,P HMBC spectrum of A2PMg in D$_2$O. 600 MHz, cryoprobe, long-range coupling constant 8 Hz, NS: 160, size of FID 32768, AQ 2.7 s. The cross peaks and $^{31}$P signals are assigned to *A2PMg* and *Imp d*. Chemical shifts δ of the $^{31}$P signals (ppm): *APMg* (1.05); *Imp d* (-2.32).

Table 1. NMR spectroscopic data of A2PMg measurements (D$_2$O, pH 7) . Multiplicity: d, doublet; t, triplet, m, multiplet; q, quartet.

| Nucleus | A2PMg | Imp a | Imp b | Imp c | Imp d | Imp e | Imp f (ethanol) | Imp g |
|---|---|---|---|---|---|---|---|---|
|  | $\delta$ (ppm) / $^3J_{C,H}$ (Hz) | | | | | | | |
| $^1H$ | | | | | | | | |
| H-4 | 4.59 (m) | | | | 4.55 (m) | | | |
| H-5 | 4.10 (m) | | | | 4.23 (m) | | | |
| H-6 | 3.76 (m) | | | | 3.74 (m) | | | |
| H-7 | | | 4.71 (q) / 7.1 | 4.12 (q) / 7.1 | 4.05 (m) | 3.66 (q) / 7.1 | 3.65 (q) / 7.1 | 3.70 (m) |
| H-8 | | 1.46 (t) / 7.2 | 1.37 (t) / 7.1 | 1.31 (t) / 7.1 | 1.25 (m) | 1.22 (t) / 7.1 | 1.18 (t) / 7.1 | 1.14 (t) / 7.1 |
| $^{13}C$ | | | | | | | | |
| C-1 | 177.2 | | | | 177.1 | | | |
| C-2 | 112.3 (d) / 5.5 | | | | | | | |
| C-3 | 175.4 | | | | 175.3 | | | |
| C-4 | 78.3 | | | | 78.5 | | | |
| C-5 | 69.6 | | | | 67.6 | | | |
| C-6 | 62.3 | | | | | | | |
| C-7 | | | 68.7 | 65.8 | 63.2 (d) / 5.8 | 66.9 | 57.4 | 67.8 |
| C-8 | | | 14.4 | 14.1 | 15.6 (d) / 5.8 | 14.0 | 16.7 | 14.6 |
| $^{31}P$ | | | | | | | | |
|  | 1.05 | | | | -2.32 | | | |

## 3.2 Measurement of the isolated A2PMg fractions

The NMR analysis of the crude A2PMg substance resulted in the structural confirmation of Imp *d* and the detection of additional ethylated impurities. However, their structures could not be elucidated due to signal overlapping and poor signal intensities. Hence, the A2PMg impurities were separated by preparative HPLC, whose fractions were concentrated by solvent evaporation. Three different fractions *1*, *2* and *3* were collected and prepared for NMR analysis.

### 3.2.1 Fractions *1* and *2*

The overlay of the $^1$H NMR spectra of fractions *1*, *2*, and crude A2PMg is shown in Fig 8. As can be seen, the protons H-4, H-5 and H-6 of A2PMg were not detected in either fraction, which was supported by missing cross peaks in the respective H,H correlation spectra.

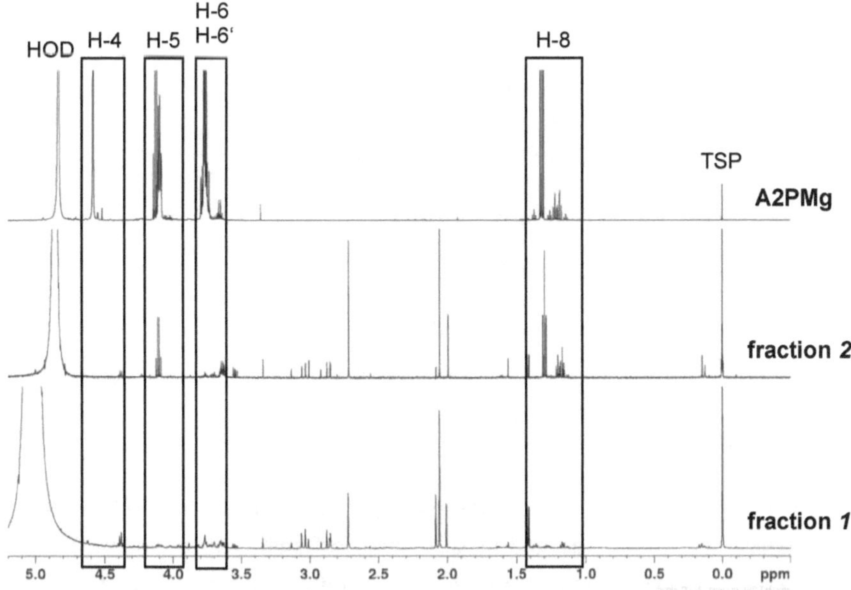


**Figure 8.** Overlay of the $^1$H NMR spectra of A2PMg, fraction *1* and *2*. The latter were recorded in $D_2O$ at pH 1. 600 MHz, cryo probe, NS: 1024 and 512, size of FID: 105818. Regions of the H-4, H-5, H-6 and H-8 protons are shown as rectangles. TSP: 3-(trimethylsilyl)propionic-2,2,3,3-$d_4$ acid sodium salt.

In both fractions *1* and *2*, several additional protons were observed in the region from δ = 1.5 - 3.5 ppm, which were not found in the crude A2PMg sample.

In fraction *2*, H-7 and H-8 protons of three ethylated impurities could be observed, which were assigned to impurities *c*, *e* and *f* (ethanol), because similar chemical shifts were observed in the A2PMg crude sample (Fig. 9). However, impurities *c* and *e* do not have an AsA structure because of missing H-4, H-5 and H-6 protons.

In fact, the spectra indicate a variety of impurities which may result from decomposition of the main impurities upon fractionation.

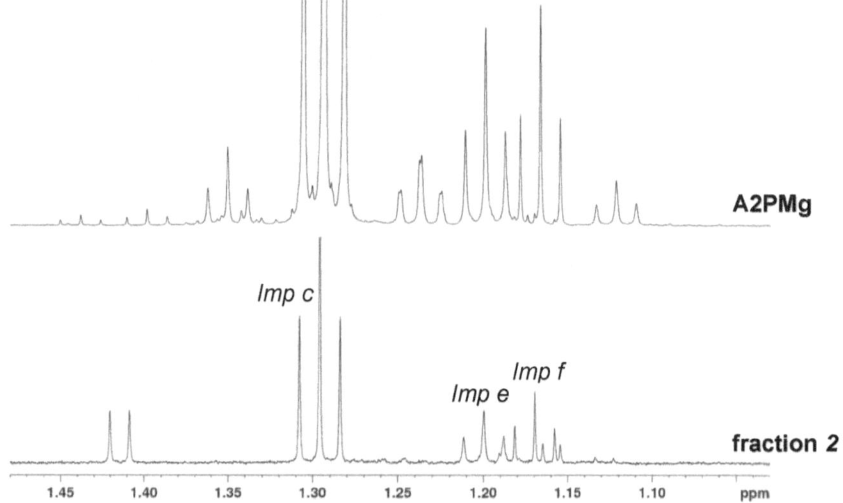


**Figure 9.** Overlay of the $^1$H NMR spectra (expanded region δ = 1.0 - 1.5 ppm) of A2PMg and fraction 2, measured in $D_2O$. 600 MHz, BBFO probe, NS: 512.

### 3.2.3 Fraction *3*

In the $^1$H NMR spectrum of fraction *3* (Fig. 10), protons belonging to an AsA structure were detected, as indicated by their chemical shifts, signal patterns, H,H and H,C correlation experiments. The protons H-7 and H-8 of the ethylated impurities *b*, *d*, *f* and *g* were also observed.

Fraction *3* revealed two additional impurities which were not observed in the crude A2PMg substance: two spin systems were identified for the protons H-4, H-5 and H-6, respectively, representing two impurities, referred to "Imp *h*" and "Imp *i*".

### 3.2.3.1 Impurity h

Imp *h* is hypothesized to be an AsA derivative which is phosphorylated on C-3 and C-5. The structure is supported by the NMR data (Tab. 2): The signals of H-4 ($\delta$ = 5.03 ppm, double doublet, $^{3}J_{\text{H-4,H-5}} \approx {}^{4}J_{\text{P-H-4}} \sim 1.79$ Hz), H-5 ($\delta$ = 4.11 ppm, multiplet) and H-6/H-6' ($\delta$ = 3.77 ppm, multiplet) could be assigned to the AsA structure of Imp *h*, which is indicated by the chemical shifts and signal patterns of those protons (Fig. 10). The H-4 signal of Imp *h* ($\delta$ = 5.03 ppm) is downfield shifted by $\Delta\delta$ = 0.5 ppm in comparison to the A2PMg substance, which might be due to decreased ionization of the 3-OH group, being a vinylogue carboxylic acid [17]. This can be explained by protonation of the acidic 3-OH group (pH of the test solution was $\sim$ 1), or its derivatization, e.g. by a phosphate ester. The chemical shifts of the H-5 ($\delta$ = 4.11 ppm) and H-6 ($\delta$ = 3.77 ppm) protons are similar to A2PMg.

**Table 2.** Proposed structure and spectroscopic data of Imp h (recorded in D$_2$O, pH 1). The curved arrows indicate the H,P couplings. Chemical shifts $\delta$ are given in ppm. dd, double doublet; m, multiplet.

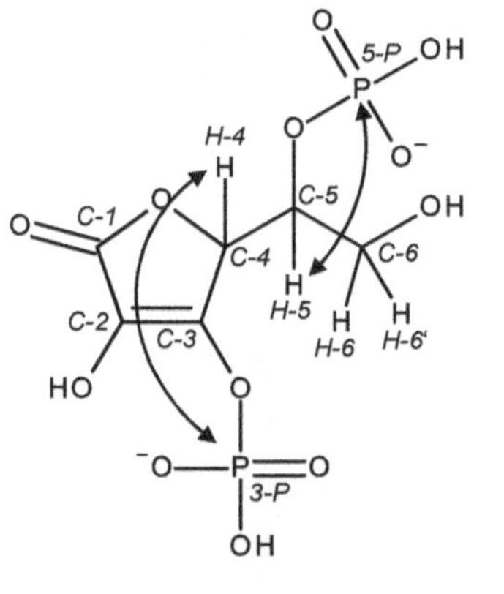

| structure | nucleus | $\delta$ (ppm) |
|---|---|---|
| | H-4 | 5.03 (dd) |
| | H-5 | 4.11 (m) |
| | H-6 | 3.77 (m) |
| | C-1 | 171.5 |
| | C-2 | 114.2 |
| | C-3 | 159.7 |
| | C-4 | 76.9 |
| | C-5 | 69.5 |
| | C-6 | 62.6 |
| | 3-P | -1.46 |
| | 5-P | 0.13 |

For Imp *h*, two cross peaks were observed in the H,P correlation spectrum (Fig. 11), indicating a coupling of H-4 and H-5 to the phosphorus at $\delta$ = -1.46 and 0.13 ppm, respectively. To assign the phosphate ester to the C-2 or C-3 position, the chemical shifts of the phosphorus signals and the splitting pattern of H-4 of A2PMg and Imp *h* were compared: the phosphorus signal of Imp *h* ($\delta$ = -1.46) was upfield shifted compared to A2PMg ($\delta$ = 1.05), which agrees with the findings reported in [9]. The

H-4 signal of Imp *h* was observed as a doublet of a doublet in contrast to the doublet in A2PMg. These differences indicate the phosphate ester of Imp *h* is located on C-3.

### 3.2.3.2 Impurity i

The structure of Imp *i* and the corresponding NMR data are shown in Tab 3. Imp *i* is assumed to be a phosphorylated AsA derivative, because similar chemical shifts and splitting patterns were observed for the signals of H-4 ($\delta$ = 4.97 ppm, doublet, $J_{H-4,H-5}$ ~ 1.79 Hz), H-5 ($\delta$ = 4.08 ppm, multiplet) and H-6/H-6' ($\delta$ = 3.76 ppm, multiplet) compared to Imp *h* (Fig. 10). The H-4 signal of Imp *i* is downfield shifted by $\Delta\delta$ = 0.4 ppm in comparison to the A2PMg substance, which might be due to the protonation of the acidic 3-OH group. A slight upfield shift could be observed for the H-5 proton of Imp *i* ($\delta$ = 4.08 ppm) compared to Imp *h* ($\delta$ = 4.11 ppm).

**Table 3.** Proposed structure and spectroscopic data of Imp i (recorded in $D_2O$, pH 1). The curved arrows indicate the H,P couplings. Chemical shifts $\delta$ are given in ppm. d, doublet; m, multiplet; n.d.: not detected (due to decomposition during storage in aqueous solution).

| structure | nucleus | $\delta$ (ppm) |
|---|---|---|
| | H-4 | 4.97 (d) |
| | H-5 | 4.08 (m) |
| | H-6 | 3.76 (m) |
| | C-1 | n.d. |
| | C-2 | n.d. |
| | C-3 | n.d. |
| | C-4 | 76.8 |
| | C-5 | 69.5 |
| | C-6 | 62.7 |
| | 5-P | -0.15 |



The H,P correlation spectrum (Fig. 11) showed one cross peak for Imp *i*, indicating a coupling of H-5 to the phosphorus at $\delta$ = -0.15 ppm. Concluding, Imp *i* is phosphorylated on C-5.

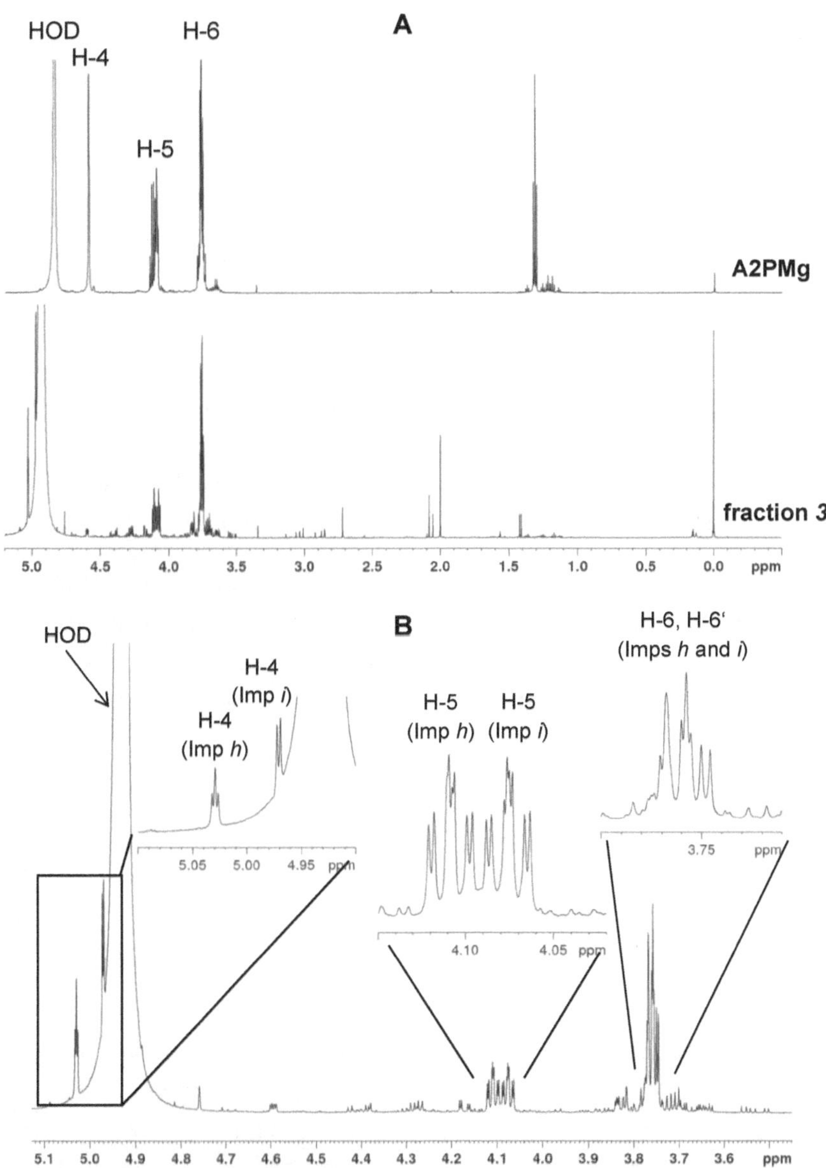



**Figure 10.** $^1$H NMR spectra of A2PMg and fraction *3*, recorded in $D_2O$ (pH 1). 600 MHz, BBFO probe, NS: 1024, size of FID: 105818, digital resolution: 0.25 Hz. (A) Spectra overlay of A2PMg and fraction *3*; (B) expanded part of the $^1$H NMR spectrum (δ = 3.5 - 5.1 ppm) of fraction *3*.

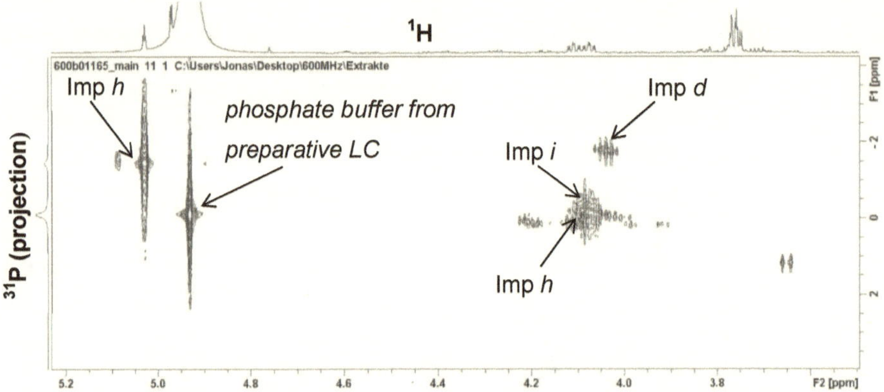


**Figure 11.** H,P HMBC spectrum of fraction *3*, recorded in $D_2O$ (pH 1). 600 MHz, BBFO probe, long range-coupling constant 8 Hz, NS: 328, size of FID: 32768. The cross peaks were assigned to impurities *d, h, i*. Chemical shifts δ of the $^{31}P$ signals (ppm) were extracted from the projected F1 axis: Imp *d* (-2.27), Imp *h* (-1.46; 0.13), Imp *i* (-0.15).

Apart from Imp *h* and *i*, the structures of impurities detected in the isolated fractions could not be elucidated due to insufficient signal intensities even with very long analysis times of > 24 h. For further structural studies, the preparation of the LC fractions has to be improved in order to increase concentration of impurities and to avoid signal overlapping in the NMR spectrum.

## 4. Conclusion

Structure elucidation of A2PMg impurities was tried using one- and multidimensional NMR spectroscopy. The crude A2PMg substance contains a mixture of ethylated impurities, including ethanol. A single impurity proposed by preceding MS analysis could be confirmed.

Several impurities detected in the A2PMg sample were found in isolated fractions from preparative LC, but could not be structurally elucidated due to poor signal intensities and overlapping. In one fraction, two additional impurities were found, which were AsA derivatives phosphorylated on C-3 and C-5 (Imp *h*), and on C-5 only (Imp *i*). Other impurities were assumed, but not confirmed, being AsA derivatives which are ethylated on the 3-, 5- or 6-OH group. Moreover, measurements indicated several ethylated compounds without AsA structure. For improved reliability, the findings should be supported with MS studies of the fractions.

# 5. References

[1] Kommentar zum Europäischen Arzneibuch, Monographie 7.0/0253 – Ascorbinsäure. 39. Aktualisierungslieferung, Wissenschaftliche Verlagsgesellschaft Stuttgart, Stuttgart, 2011.

[2] O. Arrigoni, M.C. De Tullio, Ascorbic acid: much more than just an antioxidant. Biochim. Biophys. Acta 2002, 1569, 1-9.

[3] R-I. Hata, H. Senoo, L-Ascorbic Acid 2-Phosphate Stimulates Collagen Accumulation, Cell Proliferation, and Formation of a Three-Dimensional Tissuelike Substance by Skin Fibroblasts. J. Cell. Physiol. 1989, 138, 8-16.

[4] A. Kokado, H. Arakawa, M. Maeda, New electrochemical assay of alkaline phosphatase using ascorbic acid 2-phosphate and its application to enzyme immunoassay. Anal. Chim. Acta 2000, 407, 119-125.

[5] S. Takamizawa, Y. Maehata, K. Imai, H. Senoo, S. Sato, R-I. Hata, Effects of ascorbic acid and ascorbic acid 2-phosphate, a long-acting vitamin C derivative, on the proliferation and differentiation of human osteoblast-like cells. J. Cell Biol. Int. 2004, 28, 255-265.

[6] X. Xu, M. Woźniczka, K. Van Hecke, D. Buyst, D. Mara, C. Vervaet, K. Herman, E. Wynendaele, E. Deconinck, B. De Spiegeleer, Structural study of L-ascorbic acid 2-phosphate magnesium, a raw material in cell and tissue therapy. J. Biol. Inorg. Chem. 2020, 25, 875-885.

[7] E. Cutolo, A. Larizza, Synthesis of 3-phosphoric ester of L-ascorbic acid. Gazz. Chim. Ital. 1961, 91, 964.

[8] V.M. Clark, J.W.B. Hershey, D.W. Hutchinson, The oxidative dephosphorylation of phosphoryl esters derived from L-ascorbic acid. Experientia 1966, 22, 425.

[9] C.H. Lee, P.A. Seib, Y.T. Liang, R.C. Hoseney, C.W. Deyoe, Chemical synthesis of several phosphoric esters of L-ascorbic acid. Carbohydr. Res. 1978, 67, 127-138.

[10] K. Yoshida, Y. Kawashima, Process for production of 2-phosphated esters of ascorbic acid. United States Patent No. 5,118,817, June 2, 1992.

[11] Y. Ishimura, Y. Kurata, Method for producing L-ascorbic acid 2-phosphates. United States Patent No. 5,110,951, May 5, 1992.

[12] P.A. Sieb, C.W. Deyoe, R.C. Hoseney, Method of preparation of 2-phosphate esters of ascorbic acid. United States Patent No. 4,179,445, Dec. 18, 1979.

[13] H. Nomura, T. Ishiguro, S. Murimoto, Studies on L-Ascorbic Acid Derivatives. II. L-Ascorbic Acid 3-Phosphate and 3-Pyrophosphate. Chem. Pharm. Bull. 1969, 17, 381-386.

[14] H. Nomura, T. Ishiguro, S. Morimoto, Studies on L-Ascorbic Acid Derivatives. III. Bis(L-ascorbic acid-3,3')phosphate and L-Ascorbic Acid 2-Phosphate. Chem. Pharm. Bull. 1969, 17, 387-393.

[15] H. Nomura, M. Shimomura, S. Morimoto, Studies on L-Ascorbic Acid Derivatives. VI. Phosphorylation of L-Ascorbic Acid and Its Isopropylidene Derivative. Chem. Pharm. Bull. 1971, 19, 1433-1437.

[16] H. Nomura, M. Kuwayama, T. Ishiguro, S. Morimoto, Studies on L-Ascorbic Acid Derivatives. V. Hydrolysis of L-Ascorbic Acid 3-Phosphate. Chem. Pharm. Bull 1971, 19, 341-354.

[17] B.M. Tolbert, M. Downing, R.W. Carlson, M.K. Knight, E.M. Baker, Chemistry and metabolism of ascorbic acid and ascorbate sulfate. Ann. N. Y. Acad. Sci. 1975, 258, 48-69.

[18] X. Xu, J. Urlaub, M. Woźniczka, E. Wynendaele, K. Herman, C. Schollmayer, B. Diehl, S. Van Calenbergh, U. Holzgrabe, B. De Spiegeleer, Zwitterionic-hydrophilic interaction liquid chromatography for L-ascorbic acid 2-phosphate magnesium, a raw material in cell therapy. J. Pharm. Biomed. Anal. 2019, 165, 338-345.

[19] A. Krężel, W. Bal, A formula for correlating $pK_a$ values determined in $D_2O$ and $H_2O$. J. Inorg. Biochem. 2004, 98, 161-166.

[20] J.V. Paukstelis, D.D. Mueller, P.A. Seib, D.W. Lillard Jr., NMR Spectroscopy of Ascorbic Acid and Its Derivatives In: Ascorbic Acid: Chemistry, Metabolism, and

Uses; P.A. Seib, B.M. Tolbert (Eds.), Adv. Chem. Ser. 200,. Am. Chem. Soc. 1982, 125-151.

[21] R.S. Reid, The proton NMR spectrum of ascorbic acid: A relevant example of deceptively simple second-order behavior. J. Chem. Educ. 1989, 66, 344-345.

[22] E. Pretsch, P. Bühlmann, M. Badertscher, Spektroskopische Daten zur Strukturaufklärung organischer Verbindungen, 5. Auflage, Springer, Berlin/Heidelberg, 2010.

## 3.3 Investigation of isomerization of dexibuprofen in a ball mill using chiral capillary electrophoresis

Jonas Urlaub,[1] Reinhard P. Kaiser,[1] Oliver Scherf-Clavel, Carsten Bolm, Ulrike Holzgrabe

[1]Equal contributors



**Abstract**

Beside the racemate, the $S$-enantiomer of ibuprofen (Ibu) is used for treatment of inflammation and pain. Since the configurational stability of $S$-Ibu in solid state is of interest, it was studied by means of ball milling experiments. For the evaluation of the enantiomeric composition, a chiral CE method was developed and validated according to the ICH guideline Q2(R1). The addition of $Mg^{2+}$, $Ca^{2+}$ or $Zn^{2+}$ ions to the background electrolyte (BGE) was found to improve Ibu enantioresolution. Chiral separation of Ibu enantiomers was achieved on a 60.2 cm (50.0 cm effective length) × 75 µm fused-silica capillary using a background electrolyte (BGE) composed of 50 mM sodium acetate, 10 mM magnesium acetate tetrahydrate and 35 mM heptakis-(2,3,6-tri-$O$-methyl)-β-cyclodextrin (TM-β-CD) as chiral selector. The quantification of $R$-Ibu in mixture was performed using the normalization procedure. Linearity was evaluated in the range of 0.68 - 5.49% $R$-Ibu ($R^2$ = 0.999), recovery was found to range between 97 and 103%, the RSD of intra- and interday precision below 2.5%, and the limit of quantification for $R$- in $S$-Ibu was calculated to be 0.21% (extrapolated) and 0.15% (dilution of racemic ibuprofen), respectively. Isomerization of $S$-Ibu was observed under basic conditions by applying long milling times and high milling frequencies.

# 1. Introduction

There are numerous chiral drugs on the market, which are administered as racemic mixtures, although pharmacological activity often resides in one enantiomer only. Its chiral antipode may show reduced activity, no activity at all or even toxicity. The probably most widely known example of a toxic distomer is the *S*-isomer of thalidomide showing pronounced teratogenic effects [1]. Most of the β-blockers like metoprolol and bisoprolol salts are applied as racemic mixtures, although it is known that pharmacological activity is almost exclusively ascribed to one enantiomer only [2]. The same holds true for nonsteroidal anti-inflammatory drugs (NSAIDs) such as flurbiprofen and ibuprofen [3].

Ibuprofen is an NSAID with one stereogenic center at the α carbon atom. It inhibits the cyclooxygenase providing analgesic, antipyretic and antiphlogistic effects, because it prevents the production of inflammatory prostaglandins [4,5]. Hence, ibuprofen is frequently used for the treatment of slight and moderate pain, and rheumatic diseases. The anti-inflammatory effects of Ibu can be attributed to the (+)-*S*-enantiomer (dexibuprofen), whereas (–)-*R*-Ibu is inactive (Fig. 1). Since there is a unidirectional enzymatic conversion of *R*- into *S*-Ibu *in vivo* [6-8], the racemic mixture is usually applied. However, interindividual differences in pharmacokinetics of the enantiomers might justify the use of enantiomeric pure *S*-Ibu [9,10], which was thus launched for patient's treatment also. Certainly, a compendial monograph for *S*-Ibu does not exist.

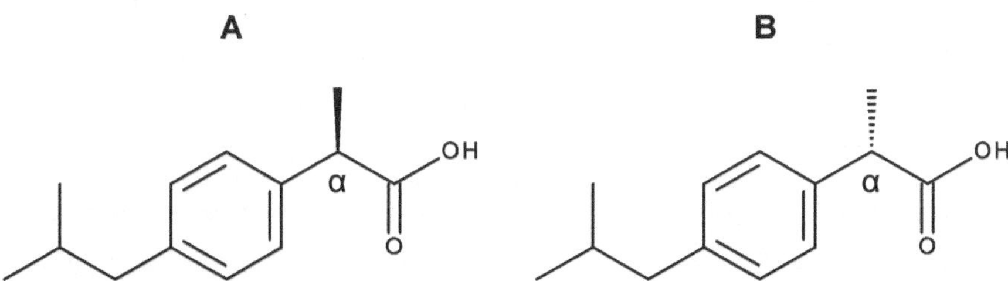



**Figure 1**. Inactive (-)-*R*-Ibu (A) and active (+)-*S*-Ibu (B).

Isomerization of *S*-Ibu was already observed *in vitro* under acidic and basic conditions, where a kinetic model of base catalyzed isomerization was evaluated [11-13]. The experiments were carried out in aqueous solution or in the melt applying high temperatures and long reaction times, including the usage of strong organic bases as isomerization additives [13]. However, the ibuprofen enantiomers were found to be highly stable under acidic conditions. Furthermore, isomerization processes in solid state have been described in the scope of asymmetric synthesis or using thermal or irradiating stress [14-19].

Mechanochemistry can offer attractive alternatives allowing a control of the reaction conditions by performing the processes in automated devices such as ball mills [20-22]. The grinding, shearing, pulling, kneading, and milling in such instruments transmits mechanical energy to reactive media inducing chemical reactions including bond-breaking and -forming processes. Many of these transformations proceed in the absence of solvent resulting in exceptionally high reactivities and leading to unusual product compositions. Recently, ball milling has been proven to be predictive for degradation processes of a drug [23]. To the best of our knowledge, mechanochemistry has not been used to investigate the isomerization of Ibu so far. Hence, the isomerization of $S$-Ibu, which was stressed in a ball mill under solid-state conditions using basic, acidic and/or liquid additives, was studied here.

For the chiral separation of racemic Ibu by means of capillary electrophoresis, many different types of buffer, chiral selectors, capillaries and electrophoretic procedures were reported [24-41]. Among the cyclodextrins, heptakis-(2,3,6-tri-$O$-methyl)-β-cyclodextrin (TM-β-CD) was used often [25-30]. Other β-CD derivatives like native β-CD [24,31,32] or sulfated β-CD [33] were also tested. Linear dextrins were found to act as chiral selectors as well, sometimes in combination with other chiral selectors [27,34-39]. Apart from oligosaccharides, enantiomeric separation of Ibu was also achieved using bovine serum albumin [34], vancomycin [40] or avidin [41] as chiral selectors.

As buffering agents, morpholinoethanesulfonic acid [24,26,27,31] or Tris/Phosphate [25,28,29,33] were frequently used in literature. In contrast, an acetate based BGE has been sparingly employed for Ibu enantioseparation in CE [31,32]. Moreover, a comprehensive method development using cations such as $Mg^{2+}$ or $Zn^{2+}$ as BGE additives has never been performed.

Up to now there is no validated CE method in literature applied on the determination of the enantiomeric purity of $S$-Ibu; reported CE methods dealing with the quantification of Ibu enantiomers are either validated [28,29,33], or tested on enantiomeric purity [37,39]. Hence, for quantitative evaluation of the *R*-Ibu content in the *S*-enantiomer after ball milling, a simple CE separation using TM-β-CD as chiral selector and a magnesium salt as cationic additive was developed and validated as an addition to other proposed CE methods and HPLC [42].

## 2. Materials and methods

### 2.1 Chemicals and reagents

Acetic acid ≥ 99.8%, HPLC grade methanol, sodium hydroxide pellets and magnesium acetate tetrahydrate ≥ 99% were obtained from Merck KGaA (Darmstadt, Germany). Calcium chloride hexahydrate ≥ 97%, magnesium chloride hexahydrate ≥ 99%, magnesium sulfate heptahydrate ≥ 99.5% and potassium chloride ≥ 99.5% were purchased from Grüssing GmbH (Filsum, Germany). Zinc sulfate heptahydrate 99.7% was obtained from VWR International (Leuven, Belgium). Hydrochloric acid 37% (m/V) for preparation of CE rinsing solution and sodium chloride ≥ 99.5% were supplied by Bernd Kraft GmbH (Duisburg, Germany). TM-β-CD ≥ 98%, HPLC grade acetonitrile, potassium hydroxide ≥ 99.95%, HPLC grade ethyl acetate ≥ 99.7%, HPLC grade water used for stress tests, hydrochloric acid 37% (m/V) as neutralizing agent and $FeCl_3$ > 97% were purchased from Sigma-Aldrich Chemie GmbH (Steinheim, Germany). Silica gel and aluminium oxide were supplied by Fisher Scientific GmbH (Schwerte, Germany). *S*- and racemic ibuprofen were kindly provided by Pen Tsao chemical industry ltd. (Hong Kong, China). Ultrapure water for CE measurements was produced by a water purification system from Merck Millipore (Darmstadt, Germany). 0.20 µm PVDF filters were supplied by Carl Roth GmbH (Karlsruhe, Germany). For filtration of reaction mixtures, Labsolute filter circles type 2020 DIN 53137 (5 - 13 µm) from Th. Geyer GmbH & Co.KG (Renningen, Germany) were used.

### 2.2 Instrumentation

Stressing experiments (20 - 30 Hz milling frequencies) were performed using a Retsch MM400 ball mill from Retsch GmbH (Haan, Germany) with a milling jar (10 mL) and milling ball (10 mm diameter) made of $ZrO_2$-Y (zirconia dioxide stabilized with yttria) or stainless steel. An IST 636 ball mill from InSolido Technologies

(Zagreb, Croatia) was used for the milling frequency of 35 Hz. For evaporation of solvents, a Heidolph Laborota 4000 rotary evaporator from Heidolph Instruments GmbH & Co.KG (Schwabach, Germany) was used.

CE separations were performed using a P/ACE MDQ capillary electrophoresis system from Beckman Coulter (Krefeld, Germany), equipped with a DAD. The fused silica capillaries purchased from BGB Analytik (Rheinfelden, Germany) were of 60.2 and 50.2 cm total length (50.0 or 40.0 cm effective length) with an i.d. of 75 and 50 µm, respectively.

## 2.3 CE procedure

The final method was carried out on a 60.2 cm (50 cm effective length) × 75 µm fused silica capillary. The optimized BGE (background electrolyte) consisted of 35 mM TM-β-CD, 50 mM sodium acetate buffer (pH 5.0) and 10 mM magnesium acetate tetrahydrate. The cartridge temperature was maintained at 27 °C and a voltage of +26 kV was applied (E = 432 V/cm, current approximately 75 µA). The detection was performed using a DAD at $\lambda$ = 202 nm (high sensitivity filter). The samples were injected hydrodynamically by applying a pressure of 3.45 kPa for 5 s on the anode side. Sample concentration was 0.6 mg/mL in 0.005 M NaOH.

New capillaries were conditioned by successively rinsing with water (1 min), 1 M NaOH (10 min), water (1 min), 2 M HCl (10 min), water (1 min) and BGE (5 min), followed by an equilibration step with the BGE at 20 kV for 30 min. Before daily measurements, the capillary was successively flushed with 1 M NaOH (3 min), 0.1 M NaOH (3 min), water (1 min) and BGE (5 min). In between measurements, the capillary was flushed with water (0.5 min), 0.1 M NaOH (6 min), water (1 min) and BGE (3 min) directly before injection. The applied pressure during rinsing steps was 138 kPa. For separation sequences, each buffer vial was used once only.

## 2.4 Stressing of *S*-Ibu

Isomerization tests were performed using *S*-Ibu in form of its free acid according to the milling processes shown in Tables S1 and S2 (n = 1, supplementary information). For each experiment, the milling jar and milling ball were of the same material: $ZrO_2$-Y for schemes **a**, **b** ,**d** - **g** or stainless steel for scheme **c**. For each milling process, the jar was loaded with 103.1 mg of *S*-Ibu (0.5 mmol) and optionally additives before milling. KOH was used as a basic additive at 2.0 molar equivalents (56 mg), and $FeCl_3$ as a Lewis acid at 0.1 molar equivalents (8.0 mg), respectively. As grinding auxiliaries, 103 mg of $SiO_2$ (1 weight equivalent) or 500 mg $Al_2O_3$ were applied.

In case of using KOH as an additive, after the milling procedure, the mixture was neutralized with an aqueous solution of 1 M HCl. The pH was checked to be 6 - 7, using pH paper (schemes **b**, **f**, **g**). Afterwards, the mixture was extracted with ethyl acetate and evaporated. If grinding auxiliaries such as $SiO_2$ or $Al_2O_3$ were applied, the extracted mixture was filtered before evaporation. The resulting powder was used for CE analysis.

### 2.5 Preparation of solutions for CE

### 2.5.1 BGE solutions

1 M sodium acetate buffer was prepared by dissolving 1.43 mL of acetic acid ≥ 99.8% in water, adjusting to the desired pH with 10 M sodium hydroxide solution and subsequent dilution to 25.0 mL with water. The 0.1 M magnesium acetate solution was prepared by dissolving 536 mg of magnesium acetate tetrahydrate in water and diluted to 25.0 mL with water. BGE stock solutions were stored at 4 °C, protected from light and used within 7 days. The final BGE was always freshly prepared by mixing the appropriate volumes of acetate buffer and magnesium acetate stock solutions, adding the required amount of the respective CD. The mixture was diluted with water to achieve the desired concentration.

### 2.5.2 Ibu solutions

Stock solutions of *S*- and racemic Ibu were prepared by dissolving 50.0 mg of the respective compound in 10.0 mL aqueous 0.05 M NaOH.

Test solutions for validation were prepared by mixing 600 µL of *S*-Ibu stock solution with varying amounts of rac-Ibu stock solution, diluting with water to 5.0 mL. For initial method development, rac-Ibu solutions were prepared by diluting a 5 mg/mL stock solution of rac-Ibu in methanol to a concentration of 0.4 mM. For the method optimization on the larger i.d. capillary, a 0.6 mg/mL *S*-Ibu solution in 0.005 M NaOH was used. All solutions were stored at 4 °C, protected from light.

The sample solutions were prepared by dissolving the respective sample in 0.005 M NaOH, resulting in a concentration of 0.6 mg/mL. Samples were vortexed and sonicated until complete dissolution. Sample measurement was conducted in randomized order in triplicates. The solutions were passed through a 0.20 µm PVDF filter and degassed prior to injection.

## 3. Results and discussion

### 3.1 Method development

According to Rawjee et al. [24], only the uncharged forms of the Ibu enantiomers are interacting with the CD as chiral selector. However, when using a neutral CD, differences in electrophoretic mobility and hence resolution are only possible if Ibu ($pK_S \approx 4.5$ [43]) is partially charged. Consequently, the buffer pH plays an important role for the resolution of the Ibu enantiomers.

The above mentioned concept was adopted for the CE method development approach, using an untreated fused silica capillary and applying the normal polarity mode (anode at the inlet). TM-β-CD was used as chiral selector because it has been proven to be well suitable for chiral recognition of the Ibu enantiomers [26]. An acetate buffer was chosen because it is suitable for ensuring a stable pH near the $pK_S$ of Ibu. The separation was initially developed on a 50.2 cm × 50 µm fused silica capillary, investigating the effects of the pH, the concentration of BGE components (buffering agent, cationic additives) and TM-β-CD on the migration time and resolution $R_S$ of the Ibu enantiomers. $R_S$ was calculated according to the equation

$$R_S = 1.18 \times (t_m 1 - t_m 2) / (w_{0.5} 1 + w_{0.5} 2) \tag{1}$$

where $t_m$ is the migration time and $w_{0.5}$ is the peak width at half height. To enhance sensitivity, the method was transferred to a 75 µm i.d. capillary, considering the adjustment of the separation parameters.

### 3.1.1 Initial method development: 50 µm i.d.

The impacts of buffer concentration and pH on enantioseparation were studied on the 50.2 cm × 50.0 µm fused silica capillary, applying a voltage of +20 kV. A solution of 0.4 mM racemic Ibu was used. To this end, 30 mM TM-β-CD were dissolved in different amounts of 1 M sodium acetate buffer of pH 4.5, 5.0, 5.5 and 5.7, respectively, then diluted with water to 1.0, 2.0 or 5.0 mL, depending on the volume needed. The resulting acetate concentrations were 25 - 175 mM. The results are summarized in Tab. 1. Ibu enantiomers could not be resolved at pH 4.5 and 5 employing buffer concentrations of 25 - 75 mM. $R_S$ values $\geq$ 1.5 within about 20 min could be obtained at pH 5.5 or 5.7 with an acetate concentration of at least 125 mM. However, the resulting high currents and Joule heating led to massive band broadening, drifting and noisy baselines.

Next, it was aimed to combine low separation currents and sufficient enantioresolution. The experiments were carried out using a BGE composed of 75 mM acetate buffer (pH 5.5) and 30 mM TM-β-CD, applying a voltage of 20 kV (E = 398 V/cm) and adding varying amounts of $Zn^{2+}$ ions. Cationic additives are known to modulate the EOF by interacting with the negatively charged capillary wall. To decrease the conductivity of the BGE, zinc sulfate heptahydrate was considered as polycationic buffer additive. The $Zn^{2+}$ concentration was varied from 1 - 10 mM and the effects on migration time, resolution and current were investigated (Tab. 2). Migration times and resolution of the Ibu enantiomers consistently increased with rising $Zn^{2+}$ concentration, while the resulting current did not change considerably. Thus, it can be concluded that adding $Zn^{2+}$ ions to the BGE is more efficient than high acetate concentrations regarding resolution and separation current. However, the $Zn^{2+}$ cations were reduced to $Zn^0$ on the cathode during separation, leading to arbitrary current distortions. Hence, cations with a smaller redox potential but similar size were considered, such as $Mg^{2+}$. 10 mM zinc sulfate heptahydrate could be replaced by the same molar amount of magnesium sulfate heptahydrate, achieving similar separation results. The separation conditions with a BGE composed of 100 mM acetate buffer pH 5.25, 15 mM $MgSO_4 \times 7H_2O$, applying a voltage of 29 kV resulted in migration times of less than 10 min for the Ibu isomers and an $R_s$ value of 2.1.

**Table 1.** Buffer and pH testing results.

| pH | Acetate (mM) | $t_m$ S-Ibu | $R_S$ | Current (µA) |
|---|---|---|---|---|
| 4.5 | 25 | 6.40 | n.a. | 9 |
|  | 50 | 8.23 | n.a. | 20 |
|  | 75 | 9.35 | n.a. | 29 |
| 5 | 25 | 6.89 | n.a. | 16 |
|  | 50 | 9.16 | n.a. | 36 |
|  | 75 | 11.05 | n.a. | 52 |
|  | 100 | 10.48 | 1.05 | 69 |
|  | 125 | 12.08 | 1.32 | 81 |
| 5.5 | 25 | 7.29 | n.a. | 20 |
|  | 50 | 9.63 | n.a. | 45 |
|  | 75 | 12.20 | 1.33 | 65 |
|  | 100 | 11.95 | 1.37 | 78 |
|  | 125 | 12.91 | 1.62 | 95 |
|  | 150 | 15.85 | 1.86 | 123 |
| 5.7 | 150 | 19.80 | 2.02 | 138 |
|  | 175 | 18.61 | 1.86 | 143 |

n.a.= not available

**Table 2.** Results of $Zn^{2+}$ concentration testing (1 - 10 mM).

| $Zn^{2+}$ (mM) | $t_m$ S-Ibu | $R_S$ | Current (µA) |
|---|---|---|---|
| 1 | 11.28 | 1.37 | 50 |
| 2.5 | 11.67 | 1.55 | 48 |
| 5 | 13.72 | 1.95 | 54 |
| 7.5 | 15.28 | 2.19 | 55 |
| 10 | 16.10 | 2.33 | 55 |

The TM-β-CD concentration was varied between 10 and 80 mM to study the impact on migration time, resolution and current. The respective results are depicted in Fig. 2. Higher TM-β-CD concentrations increased the migration times and the resolution of the Ibu enantiomers (Fig. 2A).

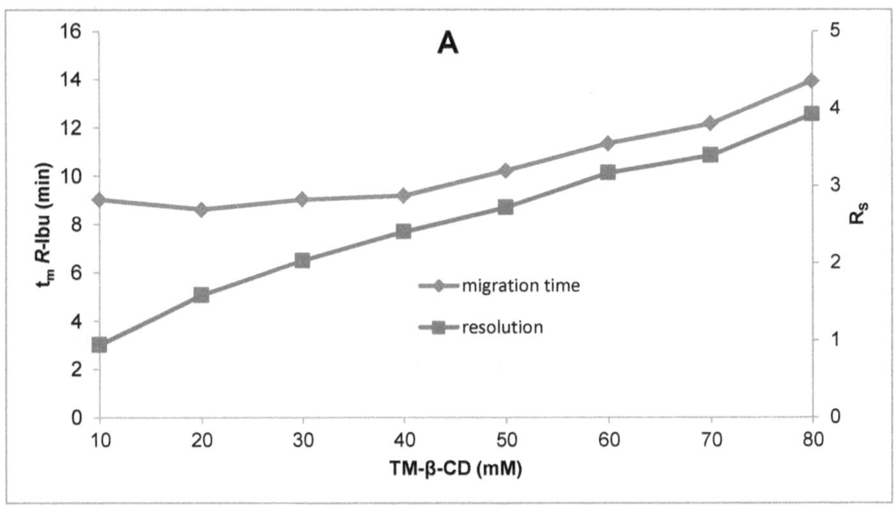


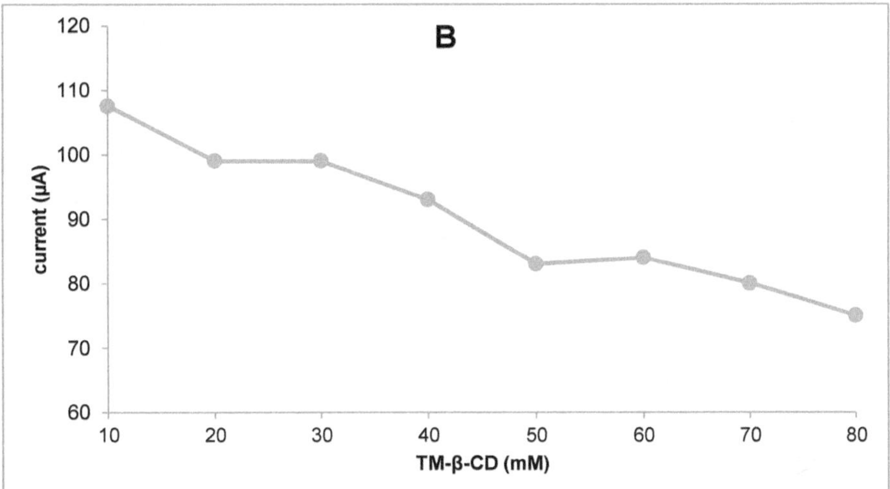


**Figure 2.** Results from TM-β-CD concentration testing (10 - 80 mM). BGE: 100 mM, sodium acetate pH 5.25, 15 mM magnesium sulfate heptahydrate. Applied voltage: +29 kV. (A) Migration times and resolution, (B) current during separation.

The current during separation decreased due to the lowering conductivity of the BGE (Fig. 2B). In fact, satisfying resolution ($R_S \geq 2$) and migration times could be achieved with TM-β-CD concentrations of 30 - 40 mM.

A detection wavelength of $\lambda = 202$ nm was chosen, even though the Ph.Eur. used $\lambda = 214$ nm in the HPLC method for the test on related substances [44], our CE method showed the highest sensitivity for detection of the *R*-isomer at $\lambda = 202$ nm.

To sum up the method development results obtained on the 50.2 cm × 50 μm capillary, sufficient separation ($R_S = 2.1$) could be achieved in less than 10 min using the above mentioned separation conditions. Current during separation was about 90 μA (E = 578 V/cm), the resulting LOQ was calculated to be 0.53% *R*- in *S*-Ibu. To further lower the LOQ, a capillary with a larger i.d. (75 μm) was used.

### 3.1.2 Method transfer and optimization: 75 μm i.d.

The method was transferred to a 50.2 cm × 75 μm capillary first (40.0 cm effective length) by reducing the voltage to 12 kV leaving the BGE unchanged, resulting in a current of about 70 μA. The long migration times of more than 30 min were reduced to 16 min by adjustment of the acetate concentration to 75 mM and $MgSO_4 \times 7H_2O$ to 15 mM, applying a voltage of 20 kV (current about 107 μA). Further studies involved the testing of organic solvents as buffer additives.

Organic solvents, e.g. methanol or acetonitrile, may affect the selectivity in CE enantioseparation of chiral drugs if added to the BGE [25,26,45,46]. As part of our method development, this was studied by adding 1 and 5% (V/V) methanol and acetonitrile to the BGE, respectively. As shown in Tab. 3, increasing amounts of the organic modifier resulted in prolonged migration times, which was more pronounced in the case of methanol compared to acetonitrile. The current during separation was slightly decreased. However, severe and irreproducible baseline shifts were observed at methanol concentrations of 5% V/V (Fig. 3). Hence, methanol and acetonitrile were withdrawn for further method development. Moreover, organic solvents were avoided for the preparation of Ibu samples because they led to noisy baselines and sample overloading effects. 0.005 M NaOH was used instead.

**Table 3.** Test results of methanol and acetonitrile as BGE additives (1 and 5% V/V).

|                     | $t_m$ S-Ibu (min) | $R_S$ | Current (µA) |
| ------------------- | ----------------- | ----- | ------------ |
| no organic solvent  | 16.23             | 2.39  | 107          |
| MeOH (% V/V)        |                   |       |              |
| 1                   | 16.41             | 2.11  | 99           |
| 5                   | 17.94             | 2.17  | 93           |
| ACN (% V/V)         |                   |       |              |
| 1                   | 16.22             | 1.94  | 104          |
| 5                   | 16.89             | 1.85  | 105          |

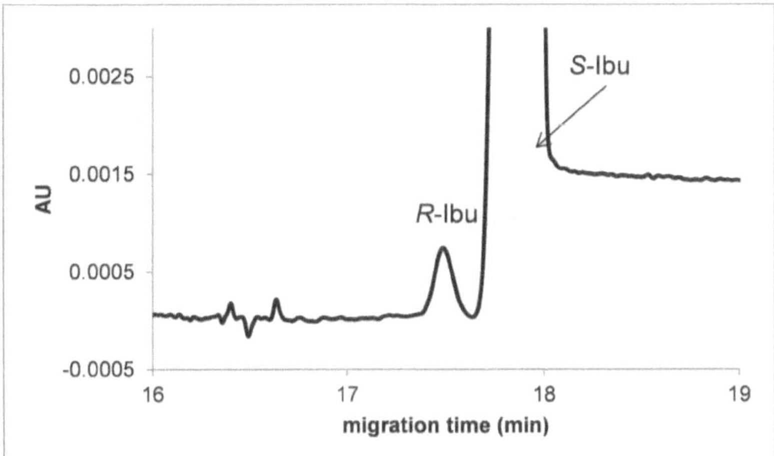


**Figure 3.** Electropherogram of S-Ibu using 5% methanol (V/V) as BGE additive.

The cationic additives magnesium, sodium and potassium salts were tested at a concentration of 12 mM and compared with respect to separation performance. Therefore, 12 mM magnesium sulfate, magnesium chloride, magnesium acetate, calcium chloride, sodium chloride or potassium chloride were added each to the BGE. The enantiomers were not resolved using NaCl or KCl. Best results regarding resolution and migration time were achieved using magnesium acetate and magnesium sulfate. Since magnesium sulfate led to noisy baselines after the S-Ibu peak, magnesium acetate was applied (Tab. 4).

**Table 4.** Testing of different cationic additives.

| Additive | $t_m$ S-Ibu (min) | $R_S$ | Current (µA) |
|---|---|---|---|
| $CaCl_2 \times 6H_2O$ | 21.14 | 2.58 | 69 |
| $MgCl_2 \times 6H_2O$ | 19.06 | 2.19 | 77 |
| $MgSO_4 \times 7H_2O$ | 17.05 | 2.08 | 83 |
| $MgAc_2 \times 4H_2O$ | 15.14 | 2.15 | 91 |
| NaCl | 13.09 | n.a. | 60 |
| KCl | 13.86 | n.a. | 64 |

Finally, a sufficient separation (migration time about 21 min, $R_S$ = 2.6) including a smooth baseline was achieved on a 60.2 cm (50.0 cm effective length) × 75 µm capillary after initial adjustment of the BGE components to 65 mM acetate pH 5.0, 12 mM $MgSO_4$ × $7H_2O$ and 35 mM TM-β-CD, applying a voltage of 20 kV (current about 70 µA).

The capillary temperature was studied as described in Tab. 5. Elevated temperatures provided faster migration times and still sufficient resolution. Best results were achieved at a temperature of 27 °C.

**Table 5.** Testing of capillary temperature.

| Temperature (°C) | $t_m$ S-Ibu (min) | $R_S$ | Current (µA) |
|---|---|---|---|
| 25 | 21.14 | 2.58 | 69 |
| 30 | 19.06 | 2.19 | 77 |
| 35 | 17.05 | 2.08 | 83 |
| 40 | 15.14 | 2.15 | 91 |

To ensure constant migration times, the rinsing procedure between each run was optimized. Rinsing schemes were tested as suggested by Wahl and Holzgrabe [47,48], where acidic, basic and organic liquids were used in varying orders upon flushing of a 60.2 cm (50.0 cm effective length) × 50 µm capillary. For our tests, the rinsing durations were adjusted accordingly. If no 0.1 M NaOH was applied as a rinsing solvent, the migration times dramatically increased, which was also observed when successively water, 0.1 M NaOH and BGE were applied. Flushing with organic solvents such as methanol followed by basic rinsing led to decreasing migration times. The optimized rinsing sequence was water (0.5 min), 0.1 M NaOH (6 min), water (1 min) and BGE (3 min). After each separation, a vial with fresh BGE was used, coping with changes such as degradation and/or electrolysis in BGE and, consequently, in separation conditions.

Injection parameters including injection duration and sample concentration were optimized to achieve the maximum sensitivity, which was determined by evaluation the $R$-Ibu peak height. The injected $S$-Ibu concentration was tested from 0.1 to 0.8 mg/mL, applying a pressure of 3.45 kPa for 4 sec at the anode side. As shown in Fig. 4, the peak height got more intense with increasing $S$-Ibu concentration, reaching a maximum at about 0.65 mg/mL. At higher concentrations, the peak height dropped because of peak broadening due to overloading effects. The resolution decreased because of the broadening Ibu peaks, but was sufficient throughout the tested concentration range ($R_S$ > 2). Along these lines, long injection times also resulted in a decrease of resolution and increase of the peak height (Fig. 5). The $S$-Ibu peak area increased linear with the tested concentration until 0.65 mg/mL, which may be indicative for beginning sample overloading at higher concentrations. Thus, preserving a safety margin, a slightly decreased $S$-Ibu concentration of 0.6 mg/mL was used.

The injection duration was varied from 3 - 10 sec at a pressure of 3.45 kPa. Fig. 5 shows a linear increase of the $R$-Ibu peak height from 4 - 10 sec, but also a severe decrease of resolution at injection durations above 5 seconds. As a compromise, the following injection parameters were chosen: a $S$-Ibu concentration of 0.6 mg/mL, which were injected for 5 sec at a pressure of 3.45 kPa. An electropherogram of $S$-Ibu (0.6 mg/mL) containing 0.68% $R$-Ibu is shown in Fig. 6. Good separation of the enantiomers ($R_S \geq 2.3$) could be achieved within about 18 min with the minor enantiomer ($R$) migrating in front of ($S$). Quantification of $R$-Ibu was performed by area normalization using the migration time corrected area $A_{corr}$ (area divided through migration time of the peak). The percentage content of $R$-Ibu was determined using

$$(A_{corr} (R\text{-Ibu}) / \sum A_{corr}) \times 100 \qquad (2)$$

The sample of $S$-Ibu provided by Pen Tsao contained a small amount of the $R$-isomer (0.68%), which can be regarded as an advantage, because it is not necessary to achieve an LOQ below 0.1% for $R$-Ibu as generally recommended by the Ph.Eur. for impurities.

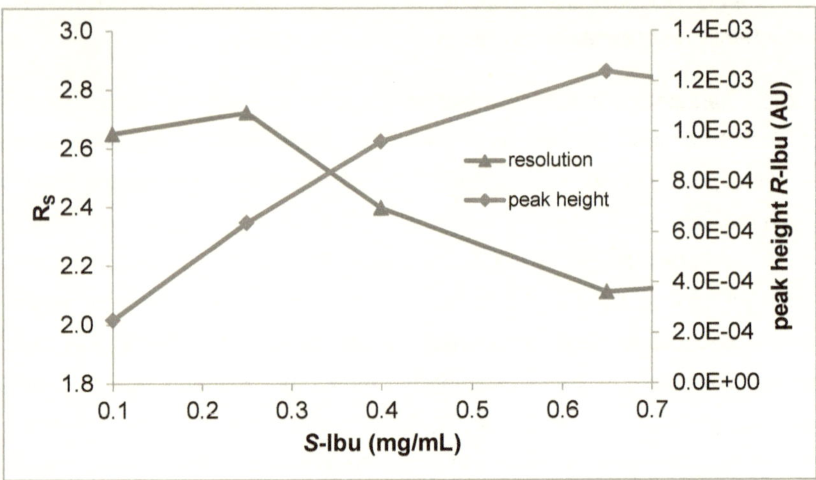


**Figure 4.** Resolution and *R*-Ibu peak height as a function of the *S*-Ibu concentration (mg/mL).

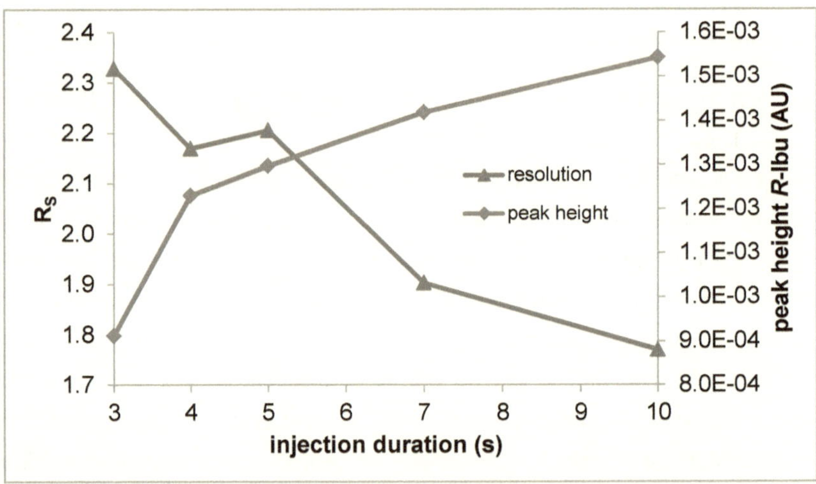


**Figure 5.** Resolution and *R*-Ibu peak height as a function of the injection duration (s).

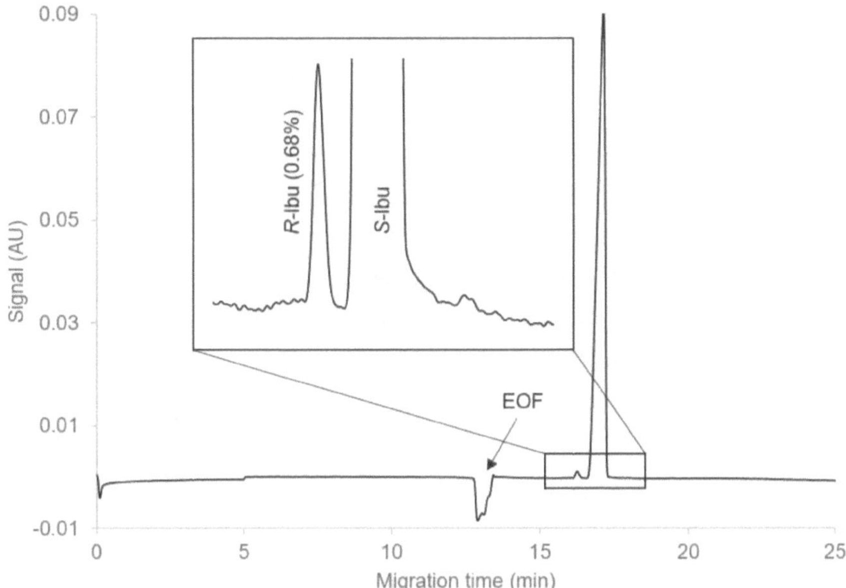


**Figure 6.** Electropherogram of the *S*-Ibu sample (0.6 mg/mL). Electrophoretic conditions: BGE: 35 mM, TM-β-CD, 50 mM, sodium acetate pH 5.0, 10 mM, magnesium acetate tetrahydrate, fused silica capillary, untreated 60.2 cm (50.0 cm from inlet to detector) × 75 µm i.d.; voltage: +26 kV; temperature: 27 °C; detection: DAD with λ = 202 nm; injection, 5.0 s at 3.45 kPa.; current: 75 µA.

## 3.2 Method validation

The validation was performed according to the ICH Guideline Q2(R1) [49]. All measurements were conducted in randomized order.

The linearity was determined at five concentration levels ranging from 0.68 to 5.49% *R*- in *S*-Ibu (y = 160.09x + 0.0705). Each concentration level was measured in triplicates. The coefficient of determination was found to be ($R^2$ = 0.9991). Accuracy was evaluated by determining the recovery ranging from 97 to 103% (Tab. S3). The small amount of *R*- in *S*-Ibu (0.68%) was taken into account by subtracting the area of the *R*-Ibu peak from the area of the *S*-Ibu peak.

The LOQ of *R*-Ibu in the presence of *S*-Ibu was determined based on a S/N of 10 by plotting the percentage *R*-Ibu against the corresponding S/N. As already mentioned, the pure *S*-Ibu sample contained 0.68% *R*-Ibu; thus the LOQ was determined by extrapolation of the calibration curve ($y = 108.59x - 12.625$; $R^2 = 0.9984$). The extrapolated LOQ was found to be 0.21% for $R$-Ibu, referring to a concentration of 1.25 µg/mL. A second approach for evaluating the LOQ of $R$-Ibu was performed by dilution of a solution of rac-Ibu until a S/N of 10 was reached and determination of the corresponding concentration of $R$-Ibu. The results are summarized in Tab. S4. The slight difference in determined LOQs pointed out in percentage $R$-Ibu (0.21 and 0.15%, respectively) may be explained by the presence of massive excess of $S$-Ibu. The comparison of the LOQs of other CE methods for the evaluation of the enantiomeric purity of $S$-Ibu (1% [37] and 0.5% [39]), revealed our method to be superior with regard to sensitivity (0.21%).

Evaluation of precision comprises repeatability and intermediate precision. The repeatability was determined by the measurement of a solution of $S$-Ibu (0.6 mg/mL) containing 0.68% $R$-Ibu ($n = 6$): an RSD of 1.52% for the $R$-Ibu content was found (Tab. S5). The RSD of the migration times was 1.31% for the $R$-Ibu and 1.46% for the $S$-Ibu peak. For intermediate precision (consecutive measurements on 2 days), with freshly prepared sample and BGE stock solutions, the RSD of the percentage $R$-Ibu content was 1.97% and of the migration times for the $R$-Ibu and the $S$-Ibu peak 2.65% and 2.78%, respectively, indicating a sufficient precision of $R$-Ibu determination.

### 3.3 Measurement of stressed $S$-Ibu samples

Fig. 7A and 7B show the CE results of isomerization after applying the milling schemes **a** - **g**. As can be seen, without the addition of KOH neither increasing the milling speed nor the reaction time leads to an isomerization of $S$-Ibu (Fig. 7A). However, a partial isomerization was observed when KOH was used. $R$-Ibu increased significantly when a combination of high milling frequency and extended milling time was applied. In particular, after a milling for 30 h at 20 Hz milling frequency, a significant isomerization was observed (samples 43, 45, 46; Fig. 7A). Only at a milling frequency of 25 Hz or higher an isomerization was already detected after 2 h of milling. To observe isomerization at a milling time of 20 min, a milling frequency of 35 Hz had to be applied (sample 39). Certain samples from milling schemes **a** and **b** were stored in solution at 4 °C for 7 days to study further isomerization (samples 21, 23, 39, 43, 44, 46). No increase in percentage $R$-Ibu could be detected, indicating an isomeric stability of *S*-Ibu in solution for at least 7 days.

Under acidic conditions, a slight isomerization was detected for sample 50 (0.80% *R*-Ibu, Fig. 7A). In contrast, sample 48 did not show any increase in the content of *R*-Ibu (0.65% *R*-Ibu) which indicates that the milling speed might be a crucial factor for isomerization for this milling scheme. No isomerization was observed in case $SiO_2$ was used as the only grinding auxiliary (scheme **d**, Fig. 7A). For milling scheme **e**, water was applied as liquid assisted grinding (LAG) agent [50] without further additives. As for schemes **a** and **d**, no isomerization could be ascertained, except for sample 57 (0.77% *R*-Ibu, Fig. 7B), where 0.1% molar equivalents of water were used. However, for sample 60, where the five-fold amount of water was employed, no isomerization was detected (0.68% *R*-Ibu). Process scheme **f** combines the usage of KOH and LAG agent. Here, only sample 72 shows minor isomerization of *S*-Ibu (0.72% *R*-Ibu, Fig. 7B). Sample 33 reveals a higher percentage of *R*-Ibu (0.80%) where no water was added. Consequently, the effect of water on isomerization of *S*-Ibu could be considered negligible. The conditions used for scheme **g** did not lead to isomerization (Fig. 7B).

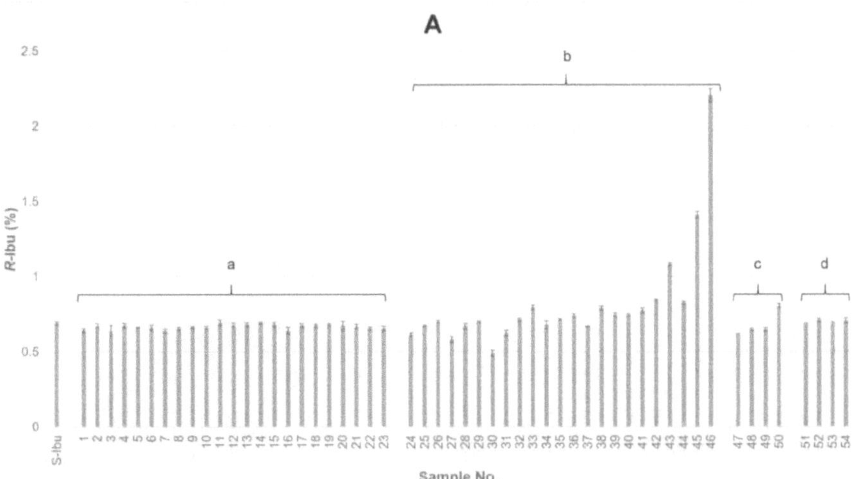

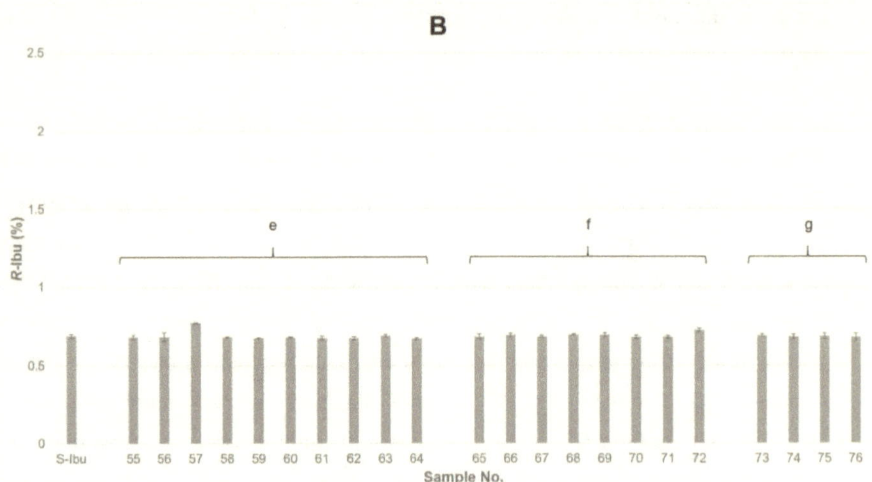

**Figure 7.** Results from isomerization tests obtained by CE measurements (n = 3). (A) Samples from scheme **a - d**, (B) samples from scheme **e - g**. For sample assignment, see Tables S1 and S2.

## 4. Concluding remarks

The CE method development revealed the addition of small cations such as $Mg^{2+}$ or $Zn^{2+}$ to highly increase the separation of Ibu enantiomers. The developed and validated CE method is proven to be capable to reliably determine the enantiomeric purity of $S$-Ibu.

To our knowledge, the isomerization of $S$-Ibu stressed in a ball mill has not been described before. The results extend the knowledge of $S$-Ibu isomerization under mechanical stress and several comparatively mild stressing conditions. Measurement results indicate that significant isomerization of $S$-Ibu only occurs on milling in presence of KOH, which gets more intense when milling time and milling speed exceed particular values. However, the extent of isomerization is limited as shown by the small increase of percentage $R$-Ibu, which emphasizes the stereochemical stability of $S$-Ibu under the conditions tested. Since a slight isomerization was only observed under basic conditions, which do not occur in tablets, capsules, and ointments, formulations are most likely stable upon storage.

*The authors thank the Wissenschaftsgemeinschaft Gottfried Wilhelm Leibniz e.V. for financial support within the "Leibniz-Forschungsprojekt PHARMSAF", and the Leibniz-Institut für Katalyse e.V. (Rostock, Germany) for collaborating in this project. Pen Tsao chemical industry ltd. (Hong Kong, China) is acknowledged for a generous gift of ibuprofen, and Natalie Fiebig is thanked for supporting method development procedures. This article was funded by the Open Access Publication Fund of the University of Würzburg which is highly appreciated.*

*The authors have declared no conflict of interest.*

## Data availability statement

The data that supports the findings of this study are available in the supplementary material of this article.

## 5. References

[1] Melchert, M., List, A., Int. J. Biochem. Cell Biol. 2007, 39, 1489-1499.

[2] Čižmáriková, R., Habala, L., Valentová, J., Markuliak, M., Appl. Sci. 2019, 9, 625.

[3] Evans, A. M., Eur. J. Clin. Pharmacol. 1992, 42, 237-256.

[4] Vane, J. R., Nature New Biol. 1971, 231, 232-235.

[5] Xie, W., Robertson, D. L., Simmons, D. L., Drug Dev. Res. 1992, 25, 249-265.

[6] Adams, S. S., Bresloff, P., Mason, C. G., J. Pharm. Pharmacol. 1976, 28, 256-257.

[7] Hutt, A. J., Caldwell, J., J. Pharm. Pharmacol. 1983, 35, 693-704.

[8] Kaiser, D. G., Vangiessen, G. J., Reischer, R. J., Wechter, W. J., J. Pharm. Sci. 1976, 65, 269-273.

[9] Davies, N. M., Clin. Pharmacokinet. 1998, 34, 101-154.

[10] Evans, A. M., Clin. Rheumatol. 2001, 20, 9-14.

[11] Xie, Y. C., Liu, H. Z., Chen, J. Y., Biotechnol. Lett. 1998, 20, 455-458.

[12] Yuchun, X., Huizhou, L., Jiayong, C., Int. J. Pharm. 2000, 196, 21-26.

[13] Ebbers, E. J., Ariaans, J. A., Bruggink, A., Zwanenburg, B., Tetrahedron Asymmetry 1999, 10, 3701-3718.

[14] Markad, S. B., Argade, N. P., J. Org. Chem. 2018, 83, 382-387.

[15] Wilson, K. R., Pincock, R. E., J. Am. Chem. Soc. 1975, 97, 1474-1478.

[16] Einhorn, C., Durif, A., Averbuch, M.-T., Einhorn, J. Angew. Chem. 2001, 40, 1926-1927.

[17] Osano, Y. T., Uchida, A., Ohashi, Y., Nature 1991, 352, 510-512.

[18] Hashizume, D., Ohashi, Y., J. Phys. Org. Chem. 2000, 13, 415-421.

[19] Sakurai, R., Suzuki, S., Hashimoto, J., Baba, M., Itoh, O., Uchida, A., Hattori, T. Miyano, S., Yamaura, M., Org. Lett. 2004, 6, 2241-2244.

[20] James, S. L., Collier, P., Parkin, I., Hyett, G., Braga, D., Maini, L., Jones, B., Friščić, T., Bolm, C., Krebs, A., Mack, J., Waddell, D. C., Shearouse, W. C., Orpen, G., Adams, C., Steed, J. W., Harris, K. D. M., Chem. Soc. Rev. 2012, 41, 413-447.

[21] Hernández, J. G., Bolm, C., J. Org. Chem. 2017, 82, 4007-4019.

[22] Friščić, T., Mottillo, C., Titi, H. M., Angew. Chem. Int. Ed. 2020, 59, 1018-1029.

[23] Buschmann, H. H., Handler, N., WIPO (PCT) world patent WO 2018/096066 A1, 2018 May 31.

[24] Rawjee, Y. Y., Staerk, D. U., Vigh, G., J. Chromatogr. 1993, 635, 291-306.

[25] Blanco, M., Coello, J., Iturriaga, H., Maspoch, S., Pérez-Maseda, C., J. Chromatogr. A 1998, 793, 165-175.

[26] Fanali, S., Aturki, Z., J. Chromatogr. A 1995, 694, 297-305.

[27] Bjørnsdottir, I., Kepp, D. R., Tjørnelund, J., Hansen, S.H., Electrophoresis 1998, 19, 455-460.

[28] Główka, F., Karaźniewicz, M., Electrophoresis 2007, 28, 2726-2737.

[29] Główka, F., Karaźniewicz, M., Anal. Chim. Acta 2005, 540, 95-102.

[30] Fillet, M., Hubert, P., Crommen, J., Electrophoresis 1997, 18, 1013-1018.

[31] Reijenga, J. C., Ingelse, B. A., Everaerts, F. M., J. Chromatogr. A 1997, 792, 371-378.

[32] Guttman, A., Electrophoresis 1995, 16, 1900-1905.

[33] Jabor, V. A. P., Lanchote, V. L., Bonato, P. S., Electrophoresis 2002, 23, 3041-3047.

[34] Sun, F., Wu, N., Barker, G., Hartwick, R. A., J. Chromatogr. A 1993, 648, 475-480.

[35] Soini, H., Stefansson, M., Riekkola, M. L., Novotny, M. V., Anal. Chem. 1994, 66, 3477-3484.

[36] D'Hulst, A., Verbeke, N., J. Chromatogr. A 1992, 608, 275-287.

[37] D'Hulst, A., Verbeke, N., Electrophoresis 1994, 15, 854-863.

[38] Nishi, H., Izumoto, S., Nakamura, K., Nakai, H., Sato, T., Chromatographia 1996, 42, 617-630.

[39] Simó, C., Gallardo, A., San Román, J., Barbas, C., Cifuentes, A., J. Chromatogr. B 2002, 767, 35-43.

[40] Armstrong, D. W., Rundlett, K. L., Chen, J. R., Chirality 1994, 6, 496-509.

[41] Tanaka, Y., Matsubara, N., Terabe, S., Electrophoresis, 1994, 15, 848-853.

[42] Bhushan, R., Martens, J., Biomed. Chromatogr. 1998, 12, 309-316.

[43] Kommentar zum Europäischen Arzneibuch, Monographie 7.0/0721 – Ibuprofen. 52. Aktualisierungslieferung, Wissenschaftliche Verlagsgesellschaft Stuttgart, Stuttgart, 2015.

[44] Council of Europe, Ibuprofen monograph No. 01/2017:0721 corrected 9.6, in: European Pharmacopoeia Online, 10th ed., EDQM, Strasbourg 2020. Available from: https://pheur.edqm.eu/subhome/10-3.

[45] Wren, S. A. C., Rowe, R. C., J. Chromatogr. A 1992, 609, 363-367.

[46] Fanali, S., J. Chromatogr. A 1991, 545, 437-444.

[47] Wahl, J., Holzgrabe, U., J. Res. Anal. 2017, 3, 73-80.

[48] Wahl, J., The Use of Ionic Liquids in Capillary Electrophoresis Enantioseparation, PhD book, Würzburg 2019, pp. 67-81. URN: urn:nbn:de:bvb:20-opus-176397.

[49] ICH Guideline Q2(R1) Validation of Analytical Procedures: Text and Methodology 1996, Geneva, Switzerland. Available from: https://www.ich.org/page/quality-guidelines.

[50] Friščić, T., Trask, A. V., Jones, W., Motherwell, W. D. S. Angew. Chem. Int. Ed. 2006, 45, 7546-7550.

## 6. Supplementary Information

**Table S1.** Stressing conditions (schemes **a** - **d**). Amounts of additives / auxiliaries used: KOH: 2 eq; $FeCl_3$: 0.1 eq; $Al_2O_3$: 500 mg; $SiO_2$: 1 weight equivalent (103 mg). "eq": molar eqivalents.

| Milling scheme | Sample No. | Milling speed (Hz) | Milling time | Additive / Auxiliary |
|---|---|---|---|---|
| a | 1 - 5 | 20 | [a] | - |
| | 6 - 10 | 25 | [a] | - |
| | 11 - 15 | 30 | [a] | - |
| | 16 - 20 | 35 | [a] | - |
| | 21[b] | 20 | 30 h | - |
| | 22 | 20 | 60 h | - |
| | 23[b] | 20 | 120 h | - |
| b | 24 - 28 | 20 | [a] | KOH |
| | 29 - 33 | 25 | [a] | KOH |
| | 34 - 38 | 30 | [a] | KOH |
| | 39[b] - 43[b] | 35 | [a] | KOH |
| | 44[b] | 20 | 30 h | KOH |
| | 45 | 20 | 60 h | KOH |
| | 46[b] | 20 | 120 h | KOH |
| c | 47 | 20 | 20 min | $FeCl_3$ |
| | 48 | 20 | 120 min | $FeCl_3$ / $Al_2O_3$ |
| | 49 | 30 | 20 min | $FeCl_3$ |
| | 50 | 30 | 120 min | $FeCl_3$ / $Al_2O_3$ |
| d | 51 | 20 | 20 min | $SiO_2$ |
| | 52 | 20 | 120 min | $SiO_2$ |
| | 53 | 30 | 20 min | $SiO_2$ |
| | 54 | 30 | 120 min | $SiO_2$ |

[a] Milling time 20, 40, 60, 90, 120 min each row

[b] Sample solutions were measured again after 7 days (stored at 4 °C)

**Table S2.** Stressing conditions (schemes **e** - **g**) with varying amounts of water as liquid assisted grinding agent. Amounts of additives / auxiliaries used: KOH: 2 eq; $SiO_2$: 1 weight equivalent (103 mg). "eq": molar equivalents.

| Milling scheme | Sample No. | Milling speed (Hz) | Milling time | Additive / Auxiliary |
|---|---|---|---|---|
| e | 55 | 25 | 20 min | $H_2O$ (0.1 eq) |
| | 56 | 25 | 120 min | $H_2O$ (0.1 eq) |
| | 57 | 25 | 20 h | $H_2O$ (0.1 eq) |
| | 58 | 25 | 20 min | $H_2O$ (0.5 eq) |
| | 59 | 25 | 120 min | $H_2O$ (0.5 eq) |
| | 60 | 25 | 20 h | $H_2O$ (0.5 eq) |
| | 61 | 25 | 20 min | $H_2O$ (1.0 eq) |
| | 62 | 25 | 120 min | $H_2O$ (1.0 eq) |
| | 63 | 25 | 20 min | $H_2O$ (10 eq) |
| | 64 | 25 | 120 min | $H_2O$ (10 eq) |
| f | 65 | 25 | 20 min | KOH / $H_2O$ (0.1 eq) |
| | 66 | 25 | 120 min | KOH / $H_2O$ (0.1 eq) |
| | 67 | 25 | 20 min | KOH / $H_2O$ (0.5 eq) |
| | 68 | 25 | 120 min | KOH / $H_2O$ (0.5 eq) |
| | 69 | 25 | 20 min | KOH / $H_2O$ (1.0 eq) |
| | 70 | 25 | 120 min | KOH / $H_2O$ (1.0 eq) |
| | 71 | 25 | 20 min | KOH / $H_2O$ (10 eq) |
| | 72 | 25 | 120 min | KOH / $H_2O$ (10 eq) |
| g | 73 | 25 | 20 min | $H_2O$ (0.1 eq) / $SiO_2$ |

**Table S2.** (Continued)

| | | | |
|---|---|---|---|
| 74 | 25 | 120 min | $H_2O$ (0.1 eq) / $SiO_2$ |
| 75 | 25 | 20 min | KOH, $H_2O$ (0.1 eq) / $SiO_2$ |
| 76 | 25 | 120 min | KOH, $H_2O$ (0.1 eq) / $SiO_2$ |

**Table S3.** Validation: accuracy (n = 3).

| *R*-Ibu added (μg) | *R*-Ibu (%) | Recovery (%) | RSD (%) |
|---|---|---|---|
| 2.47 | 0.77 | 101 | 1.60 |
| 4.94 | 0.87 | 103 | 1.24 |
| 49.5 | 2.35 | 100 | 0.30 |
| 86.7 | 3.61 | 101 | 0.25 |
| 111.4 | 4.31 | 97 | 0.47 |
| 149.0 | 5.49 | 97 | 0.53 |

**Table S4.** Validation: LOQ of *R*-Ibu.

| *Extrapolation (Calibration curve)* | | | | |
|---|---|---|---|---|
| *R*-Ibu (%) | 0.68 | 2.35 | 3.61 | 4.31 | 5.49 |
| S/N | 68.7 | 238 | 370 | 453 | 593 |

LOQ (S/N = 10, extrapolated): 0.21% ($\triangleq$ 1.25 μg/mL)

$y = 108.59x - 12.625$; $R^2 = 0.9984$

| *Dilution of rac-Ibu solution* | | | | |
|---|---|---|---|---|
| *R*-Ibu (μg/mL) | 0.25 | 0.49 | 0.74 | 0.99 | 1.23 |
| S/N | 3.1 | 5.0 | 7.7 | 10.9 | 13.6 |

LOQ (S/N = 10): 0.92 μg/mL ($\triangleq$ 0.15%)

$y = 10.943x - 0.029$; $R^2 = 0.9928$

**Table S5**. Validation: precision (n = 6); $t_m$ = migration time.

| Repeatability | Run | 1 | 2 | 3 | 4 | 5 | 6 | RSD (%) |
|---|---|---|---|---|---|---|---|---|
| Day 1 | $R$-Ibu (%) | 0.69 | 0.68 | 0.67 | 0.66 | 0.69 | 0.68 | 1.52 |
| | $t_m$ $R$-Ibu (min) | 16.2 | 16.2 | 16.7 | 16.7 | 16.6 | 16.5 | 1.31 |
| | $t_m$ $S$-Ibu (min) | 17.1 | 17.1 | 17.6 | 17.7 | 17.5 | 17.4 | 1.46 |
| Day 2 | $R$-Ibu (%) | 0.66 | 0.68 | 0.68 | 0.66 | 0.65 | 0.69 | 2.21 |
| | $t_m$ $R$-Ibu (min) | 15.9 | 15.6 | 16.0 | 17.3 | 16.1 | 16.1 | 3.46 |
| | $t_m$ $S$-Ibu (min) | 16.8 | 16.4 | 16.9 | 18.2 | 17.0 | 17.0 | 3.55 |
| Interday precision | $R$-Ibu (%) | | | | | | | 1.97 |
| | $t_m$ $R$-Ibu (min) | | | | | | | 2.65 |
| | $t_m$ $S$-Ibu (min) | | | | | | | 2.78 |

## 3.4 Degradation profiling of Clopidogrel hydrogen sulfate stressed in the solid state using mechanochemistry under oxidative conditions

## 1. Introduction

Comprehensive stability and stress tests are integral parts of the drug approval process. As a result, the drug's stability and thus shelf life has to be determined. Of note, degradants of the respective active pharmaceutical ingredient (API) may exhibit toxic potential, and should be evaluated to ensure high safety upon drug administration. Stability indicating studies are usually conducted for 6 (intermediate and accelerated) and 12 months (long term) under specified conditions regarding humidity and temperature as prescribed by the international conference on harmonization (ICH) guideline Q1A(R2) [1]. Forced degradation studies can be considered as a less time consuming approach under more severe conditions. The aim is to identify potential degradation products (DPs) and degradation pathways of the drug compound. The Q1A(R2) guideline mentions photolysis, hydrolysis and oxidation as useful parts of the stress testing, but does not provide detailed information about the practical aspects of the forced degradation studies. Hence, some suggestions were made on how to perform them [2]. For example, hydrolysis and oxidation are commonly tested in aqueous environment using 0.1 M HCl or 0.1 M NaOH and 3% hydrogen peroxide, respectively. The photostability testing is regulated by the ICH guideline Q1B [3].

An alternative for stress testing approaches is solid state mechanochemistry. It proved to be a powerful tool in organic synthesis due to its high effectiveness and versatility without (nominal) use of solvents. The mechanical energy transferred to the reagents causes molecule transformations by altered, improved or even new reactivities and products [4-6]. Moreover, solid state mechanochemistry has been shown to be applicable for the prediction of degradation pathways of drugs. In brief, the drug compound is stressed with solid acidic, basic or oxidizing catalysts, which is conducted in an active reaction container (e.g. a ball mill), transferring chemically stimulating energy to the mixture. This approach might be superior to common stress tests carried out in solution, because the simulation of the reaction conditions in solid state results in more realistic data upon specification of shelf-life limits or storage conditions [7]. Reliable results can be achieved in a short time of a few hours under optimized conditions, which has been demonstrated on the antiplatelet drug Clopidogrel (CLP) [7].

CLP is used for the treatment of peripheral arterial disease, acute coronary syndromes and the prevention of thromboembolic events [8]. The antiplatelet activity is caused by the irreversible inhibition of the adenosine diphosphate (ADP) receptors localized on the thrombocytes [9,10]. CLP is a prodrug, which is converted into the active thiol metabolite *in vivo* by several hepatic CYP450 enzymes (Fig. 1) [8,11]. However, only the (S)-enantiomer shows antiplatelet potential [11]. It is therapeutically used as the hydrogen sulfate salt for instance.

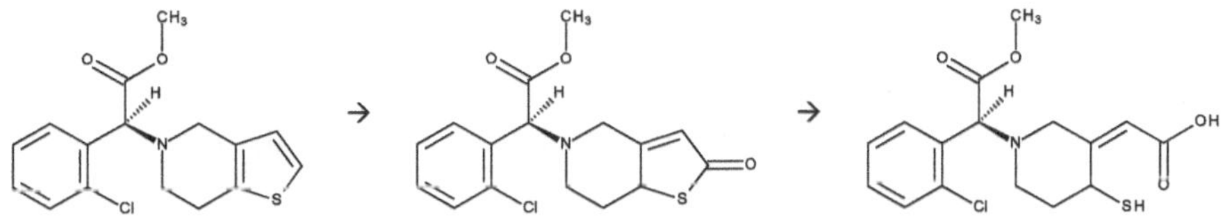

**Figure 1.** CYP450 dependent metabolic activation of (S)-CLP. The CLP prodrug is converted into 2-oxo-CLP and the active thiol derivative which interacts with the ADP receptor.

For the analysis of CLP impurities, methods based on reversed-phase liquid chromatography (RP-LC) were already reported [12-19]. Several stressing conditions including acidic, basic, oxidative, photolytic and/or thermolytic environment were applied to form and subsequently identify various CLP degradation products [13-18]. In the European Pharmacopoeia (Ph.Eur.) monograph of CLP hydrogen sulfate, the test on related substances is also performed using RP-LC, which is not compatible with mass spectrometric detection due to the usage of sodium pentanesulfonate and phosphoric acid as mobile phase additives [20].

This study describes the analysis of various degradation products of CLP which were formed under oxidative conditions in the solid state applying mechanochemistry. For structure confirming and elucidation, HPLC-MS/(MS) experiments were performed.

## 2. Experimental section

### 2.1 Chemicals and reagents

Clopidogrel hydrogen sulfate for stress tests was kindly provided by Pen Tsao chemical industry ltd. (Hong Kong, China). Clopidogrel hydrogen sulfate for method validation (certified reference substance) was purchased from Sigma-Aldrich Chemie GmbH (Steinheim, Germany). HPLC grade formic acid (FA) 99% and sodium sulfate (analytical grade) were purchased from Grüssing GmbH (Filsum, Germany), HPLC grade acetonitrile from Sigma-Aldrich Chemie GmbH (Steinheim, Germany). LC-MS grade water and LC-MS grade acetonitrile were obtained from Merck KGaA (Darmstadt, Germany). LC-MS grade formic acid ≥ 99% was purchased from VWR International (Leuven, Belgium). Ultrapure water for HPLC-UV measurements was produced by a water purification system from Merck Millipore (Darmstadt, Germany). 0.20 µm PVDF filters were purchased from Carl Roth GmbH (Karlsruhe, Germany). Oxone was supplied by the Leibniz-Institut für Katalyse e.V. (Rostock, Germany).

### 2.2 Apparatus and equipment

HPLC-UV experiments were conducted on an Agilent 1100 modular liquid chromatographic system equipped with an online vacuum degasser, a binary pump, an auto sampler, a diode array detector (DAD) and an Agilent 1200 column oven (Agilent Technologies, Waldbronn, Germany). The chromatograms were evaluated using the Agilent ChemStation® software (Rev B.03.02).

HPLC-MS experiments were carried out on a Shimadzu LCMS-2020 Single Quad instrument, using the LabSolutions software (batch 15.10.2020). Both software and instrument were from Shimadzu Deutschland GmbH, Duisburg, Germany.

HPLC-MS/MS measurements were conducted on an Agilent 1200 chromatographic system coupled to an Agilent 6460 Triple Quad LC/MS instrument (Agilent Technologies, Waldbronn, Germany). For instrument control, data collection and analysis, the Agilent MassHunter software (version B.08.00) was used.

The samples were centrifuged in a Hettich EBA 12 centrifuge (Andreas Hettich GmbH & Co. KG, Tuttlingen, Germany).

## 2.3 Stressing of CLP samples

The CLP stressing tests were conducted by the Leibniz-Institut für Katalyse e.V. (Rostock, Germany). An overview of the stressing procedure of the CLP samples in the solid state is given in Tab. 1. As the oxidizing catalyst, oxone ($KHSO_5 \times 0.5KHSO_4 \times 0.5K_2SO_4$) was either chemically adsorbed to $SiO_2$ particles ("oxone *on* $SiO_2$") at varying mass concentrations or a physical mixture of oxone and $SiO_2$ was used ("oxone *and* $SiO_2$", sample 10). Also, $SiO_2$ without further additives (sample 11) and $KNO_3$ on $SiO_2$ (sample 12) were employed as catalysts. The catalyst mixture was tested in varying amounts. The milling jar and ball material consisted of $ZrO_2$ and stainless steel, respectively. For each milling experiment, the reaction jar and the milling ball were of the same material.

**Table 1.** Treatment of the CLP samples for oxidative solid state stress tests. The milling time was 5h, except for sample 12 (10 min).

| Sample I.D. | CLP (mg) | Type of catalyst | Amount of catalyst (mg) | Jar material | Milling frequency (Hz) |
|---|---|---|---|---|---|
| 1 | 200 | oxone on $SiO_2$ (w=10%) | 730 | $ZrO_2$ | 30 |
| 2 | 200 | oxone on $SiO_2$ (w=10%) | 730 | steel | 30 |
| 3 | 200 | oxone on $SiO_2$ (w=10%) | 365 | $ZrO_2$ | 30 |
| 4 | 200 | oxone on $SiO_2$ (w=10%) | 365 | steel | 30 |
| 5 | 200 | oxone on $SiO_2$ (w=10%) | 1460 | $ZrO_2$ | 30 |
| 6 | 200 | oxone on $SiO_2$ (w=10%) | 1460 | steel | 30 |
| 7 | 200 | oxone on $SiO_2$ (w=2%) | 1460 | $ZrO_2$ | 30 |
| 8 | 200 | oxone on $SiO_2$ (w=2%) | 1460 | steel | 30 |
| 9 | 100 | oxone on $SiO_2$ (w=2%) | 730 | $ZrO_2$ | 25 |
| 10 | 100 | oxone and $SiO_2$ (w=2%) | 730 | $ZrO_2$ | 25 |
| 11 | 100 | $SiO_2$ | 730 | $ZrO_2$ | 25 |
| 12 | 100 | $KNO_3$ on $SiO_2$ (w=9%) | 275 | $ZrO_2$ | 25 |

## 2.4 Chromatographic procedure

### 2.4.1 HPLC-UV method optimization and validation

The HPLC conditions were based on the method proposed by Mashelkar and Renapurkar [14]. The optimized method was carried out on an Agilent Zorbax Eclipse Plus C8 column (double-endcapped, carbon load 7%, 250 × 4.6 mm, 5 µm particles). The mobile phases A and B were water and acetonitrile, respectively, both containing 0.1% formic acid (V/V), respectively. The gradient elution was performed as follows: 0 - 10 min: 20% B, 10 - 40 min: 20→80% B, 40 - 45 min: 80% B, 45 - 48 min: 80→20% B, 48 - 50 min: 20% B, at a constant flow rate of 1 mL/min. The injection volume was 15 µL, the temperature during separation was maintained at 25 °C. The detection wavelength was $\lambda$ = 235 nm.

For validation according to the ICH guideline Q2(R1) [21], a CLP stock solution of 5 mg/mL was prepared in a solvent mixture of mobile phase A and B (80:20 V/V) and diluted with solvent mixture to achieve the desired CLP concentration. Linearity was evaluated within the working range of 100 - 1000 µg/mL at five approximately equidistant concentrations. Intra- and interday precision were determined by measuring CLP concentrations of 100, 500 and 1000 µg/mL on two consecutive days. Accuracy was evaluated by spiking a sample with known concentrations of CLP and determining the recovery. The determination of the limit of detection (LOD) and the limit of quantification (LOQ) was based on a signal-to-noise ratio (S/N) of 3 and 10, respectively, by measuring a diluted CLP solution of known concentration. The noise was determined from a chromatogram of a blank solution over the distance of 5 times the width at half-height of the CLP peak as described in the Ph.Eur. [22]. The stability of a CLP test solution was determined, which was stored for 6 days at 4 °C, protected from light. All validation measurements were performed in triplicates.

### 2.4.2 Sample preparation and measurement

#### 2.4.2.1 HPLC-UV analysis of stressed CLP samples

The sample was weighed according to Tab. 2 and suspended in 2 mL of a mixture of mobile phase A and B (80:20 V/V), resulting in even CLP concentrations of 1 mg/mL regarding the pre-stressing conditions described in Tab. 1 (1 mg/mL CLP equivalents).

**Table 2.** Concentrations of stressed CLP samples (CLP + catalyst) employed for HPLC-UV analysis resulting in 1 mg/mL CLP equivalents.

| Sample ID | 1 | 2 | 3 | 4 | 5 | 6 | 7 | 8 | 9 | 10 | 11 | 12 |
|---|---|---|---|---|---|---|---|---|---|---|---|---|
| Sample concentration (mg/mL) | 4.65 | 4.65 | 2.83 | 2.83 | 8.3 | 8.3 | 8.3 | 8.3 | 8.3 | 8.3 | 8.3 | 3.75 |

The suspension obtained was subsequently vortexed for a few seconds and centrifuged at 10000 rpm ($g = 9320$ m/s$^2$) for 5 minutes. The supernatant was transferred into an HPLC vial for measurement, using the original HPLC method [14]. The chromatograms were compared with respect to the CLP decomposition and the formation of various degradations products using UV/Vis detection.

### 2.4.2.2 HPLC-MS analysis of stressed CLP samples

LC-MS (single quad) analysis was performed with the original HPLC method by Mashelkar et al. Prior to measurements, the samples were filtered through a 0.2 μm PVDF filter after centrifugation. Concentrations of 0.5 mg/mL CLP equivalents were used. For determination of the m/z, the total ion chromatogram (TIC) was analyzed. The ESI mode was applied in the positive scan mode with an interface temperature and voltage of 350 °C and 4500 V, respectively. The nebulizing gas flow was 1.5 L/min and the scan speed was 15000 u/s.

### 2.4.2.3 HPLC-MS/MS analysis of stressed CLP samples

HPLC-MS/MS measurements were carried out using the optimized HPLC method. For product ion and full scans on the triple quad instrument, equivalent CLP concentrations of 0.1 μg/mL and 1 μg/mL were used, respectively. The samples were filtered through a 0.2 μm PVDF filter after centrifugation. The injection volume was 2 μL. An electrospray ionization interface in the positive mode with a spray voltage of 4000 V and a gas temperature at 350 °C (flow = 10 L/min) was used. The nebulizer was set to 55 psi, the sheath gas heater to 400 °C and the sheath gas flow to 12 L/min. Experiments were carried out applying different collision energies of 10 and 30 eV (fragmentor voltage was 135 V) for precursor and product ion detection. The results were compared to the decomposition products found in the literature.

### 2.4.3 Relative response factors and LOQ/LOD of the DPs

The relative response factors (RRF) of the DPs were estimated by considering their normalized UV/Vis spectra and molar masses compared to CLP. This was accomplished by relating the absorbances at the detection wavelength $\lambda = 235$ nm of the normalized UV/Vis spectra and the molar masses of the DPs and CLP, according to the equation

$$RRF = \frac{M_{r\,(CLP)}}{M_{r\,(DP)}} \cdot \frac{A_{\lambda=235\,nm\,(DP)}}{A_{\lambda=235\,nm\,(CLP)}} \qquad (1)$$

where $M_r$ represents the molar mass and A the absorbance of the substance at $\lambda = 235$ nm in the normalized UV/Vis spectrum. If $M_r$ of the DP was not known, a molar mass ratio was assumed to be 1.

For the estimation of the LOD and LOQ of the DPs, their S/N ratios were evaluated from a chromatogram of a representative stressed sample and extrapolated to 3 (LOD) and 10 (LOQ). The corresponding concentration was calculated using the normalized areas of the DP peaks, to which the correction factors (CF, reciprocal of RRF) were applied.

## 3. Results and discussion

Parameters including injection volume, composition of mobile phases, gradient elution settings and detection wavelength were adjusted to achieve sufficient separation efficiency.

### 3.1 HPLC-UV method optimization

Several stability-indicating HPLC methods for the separation of CLP and its DPs were already described in the literature. The methods developed by Mashelkar and Renapurkar [14], Mitakos and Panderi [15] and Raijda et al. [16] were tested on a stressed CLP sample in order to achieve the best separation results. The method described by Mashelkar revealed to achieve a suitable separation of all DPs obtained by the new stress tests. The stressed CLP sample 8 (see Tab. 1) was chosen as a representative test substance because the respective chromatogram showed partially not separated peaks.

To avoid contamination of the mass spectrometer, the mobile phase additive trifluoroacetic acid (TFA) was replaced by the same amount of formic acid, which was added to both mobile phases A and B (shortened as A and B in the following). As a result, the pH of the aqueous phase (A) changed from 1.9 (0.1% TFA V/V) to 2.65 (0.1% FA V/V), which did not have a considerable influence on the separation. The flow rate and the column temperature were kept constant at 1 mL/min and 25 °C, respectively. The injected sample concentration was increased from 400 µg/mL to 1000 µg/mL CLP equivalents to obtain higher peak intensities of the impurites.

To cope with the unsatisfactory resolution of the peaks eluting in the time range from 10 - 15 min, the elution strength of the original method was lowered in this retention time window by decreasing the percentage amount of acetonitrile (B). As a result, good separation occurred when the amount of acetonitrile (B) was decreased to 25 - 20% V/V. The optimal gradient settings were applied as follows: 0 - 10 min: 20% B, 10 - 40 min: 20→80% B, 40 - 45 min: 80% B, 45 - 48 min: 80→20% B, 48 - 50 min: 20% B. The solvent mixture for sample dissolution was changed to the gradient starting conditions (80:20 A:B V/V), the injected sample volume was decreased from 20 to 15 µL. A representative chromatogram of sample 8 recorded with the original and the final method is shown in Fig. 2. The absence of matrix peaks was confirmed by spiking a blank (solvent mixture) and sample 8 with $Na_2SO_4$ or oxone at respective concentrations of 1 mg/mL.

**A**

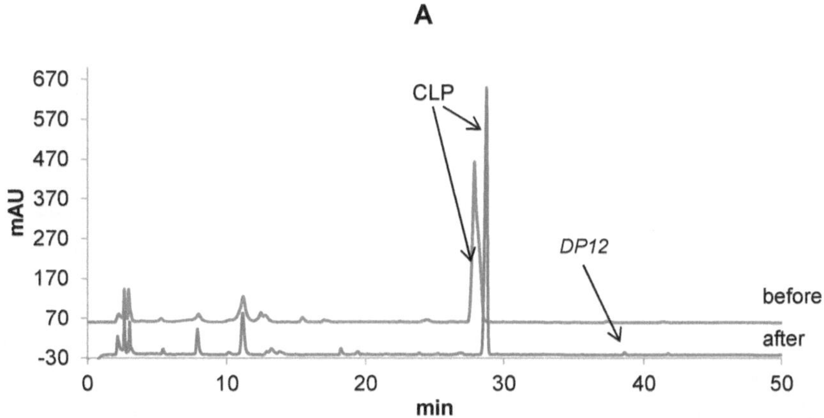

**B**

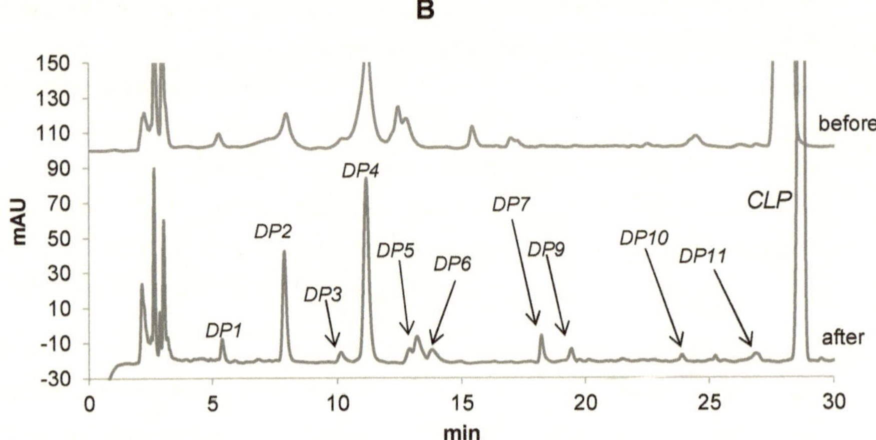



**Figure 2.** Overlay of the chromatograms of sample 8 obtained with the original method ("before") [14] and after optimization ("after"). The HPLC conditions are described in [14] and in the text, respectively. (A) Full chromatogram; (B) enlarged part. DP: degradation product. $T_R$ (min): DP1 (5.4); DP2 (7.9); DP3 (9.9); DP4 (11.2); DP5 (12.9); DP6 (13.4); DP7 (18.1); DP9 (19.4); DP10 (24.6); DP11 (26.9); CLP (28.0); DP12 (38.6); DP8 (expected at about 18.5 min) was not detected in sample 8.

## 3.2 Method validation

The optimized HPLC-UV method was validated according to ICH Q2(R1). The linearity was confirmed within the tested concentration range from 100 - 1000 µg/mL ($y = 17.227x + 100.78$, $R^2 = 0.9999$, Tab. 3).

**Table 3.** Validation data: linearity (n = 3).

| CLP concentration (µg/mL) | Average peak area (mAU) | RSD (%) |
|---|---|---|
| 100 | 1767 | 0.27 |
| 300 | 5229 | 0.66 |
| 500 | 8761 | 0.35 |
| 700 | 12084 | 0.13 |
| 1000 | 17186 | 0.22 |

The method precision was tested on two consecutive days (intra- and interday precision) at three concentration levels (100, 500 and 1000 µg/mL), resulting in an RSD of < 0.5 and < 1%, respectively (Tab. 4).

**Table 4.** Validation data: intra- and interday precision (n = 3).

| | Intraday precision | | Interday precision | |
|---|---|---|---|---|
| CLP concentration (µg/mL) | Average peak area (mAU) | RSD (%) | Average peak area (mAU) | RSD (%) |
| 100 | 1767 | 0.27 | 1772 | 0.57 |
| 500 | 8761 | 0.35 | 8775 | 0.66 |
| 1000 | 17186 | 0.22 | 17253 | 0.46 |

The accuracy was evaluated by determining the recovery of CLP, which was spiked with 100, 250 and 500 µg/mL at the stressed sample 6. The data in Tab. 5 show the resulting recoveries ranging from 103.6 - 104.5% (mean value 104.1%, RSD < 0.25%).

**Table 5.** Validation data: accuracy (n = 3).

| Spiked CLP concentration (µg/mL) | Recovery (%) | RSD (%) |
|---|---|---|
| 100 | 103.6 | 0.22 |
| 250 | 104.1 | 0.21 |
| 500 | 104.5 | 0.13 |

The LOD and LOQ of CLP were established by diluting a CLP solution of known concentration until the signal-to-noise ratio (S/N) reached 3 and 10, respectively. For 15 µL injection volume, the LOD was 0.46 µg/mL and the LOQ was 1.36 µg/mL.

The stability of a 1000 µg/mL CLP solution was tested, which was stored in a refrigerator at 4 °C for 6 days. The resulting CLP content was found to be slightly decreased by 0.5% (RSD 0.049%), which was considered neglectable for sample measurement because the samples were used within 24 hours after preparation.

### 3.3 HPLC measurement of stressed samples

The HPLC-UV measurement results of the stressed CLP samples are summarized in Fig. 3. The amounts of remaining CLP and formed DPs were evaluated using the normalization procedure.

As depicted in Fig. 3, the samples milled in a steel jar showed more intense CLP degradation than their counterparts treated in a $ZrO_2$ mill. No influence of the amount of the catalyst mixture added to the CLP drug substance was detected. However, a higher $SiO_2$-oxone-ratio of the catalyst led to increased degradation (samples 6 and 8). This finding does not seem plausible at first glance, because a higher amount of oxidizing catalyst is expected to decompose the API more intensely. Additionally, the degradation profiles of samples 1 - 6 (10% oxone m/m) are very similar, whereas the samples 7 - 10 (2% oxone m/m) showed a substantially increased formation of *DP4*. Interestingly, sample 10 does not show more degradation than sample 9, but also a different degradation profile. This finding points to the difference between chemically adsorbed oxone on $SiO_2$ and the simple physical blend. Even though no oxidizing agent was used for the stressing of sample 11, a distinct degradation was observed, which may be due to the mechanical energy transmitted. A milling frequency of 30 Hz (sample 7) led to slightly enhanced degradation compared to 25 Hz (sample 9).

The usage of $KNO_3$ as oxidizing agent resulted in a CLP degradation of approximately 70% (sample 12). In contrast to the other samples, a high amount of *DP2*, *DP7*, and other unknown impurities were formed. The UV spectra recorded within this region indicated the presence of *DP5* and *DP6*. The respective chromatogram is shown in Fig. 4. For better reliability of the results, the sample measurement should be repeated using the optimized HPLC-UV conditions.

Degradation profiling of Clopidogrel hydrogen sulfate stressed in the solid state using mechanochemistry under oxidative conditions

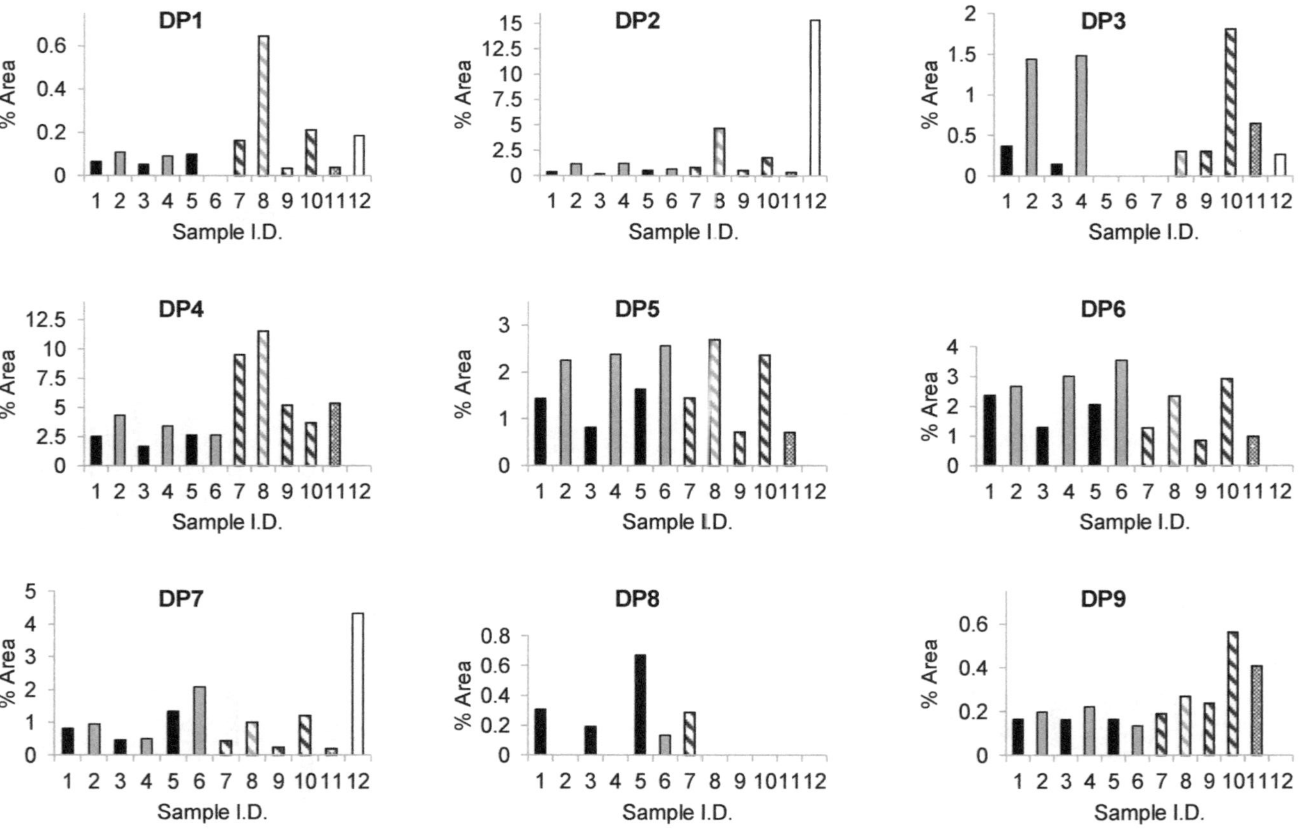

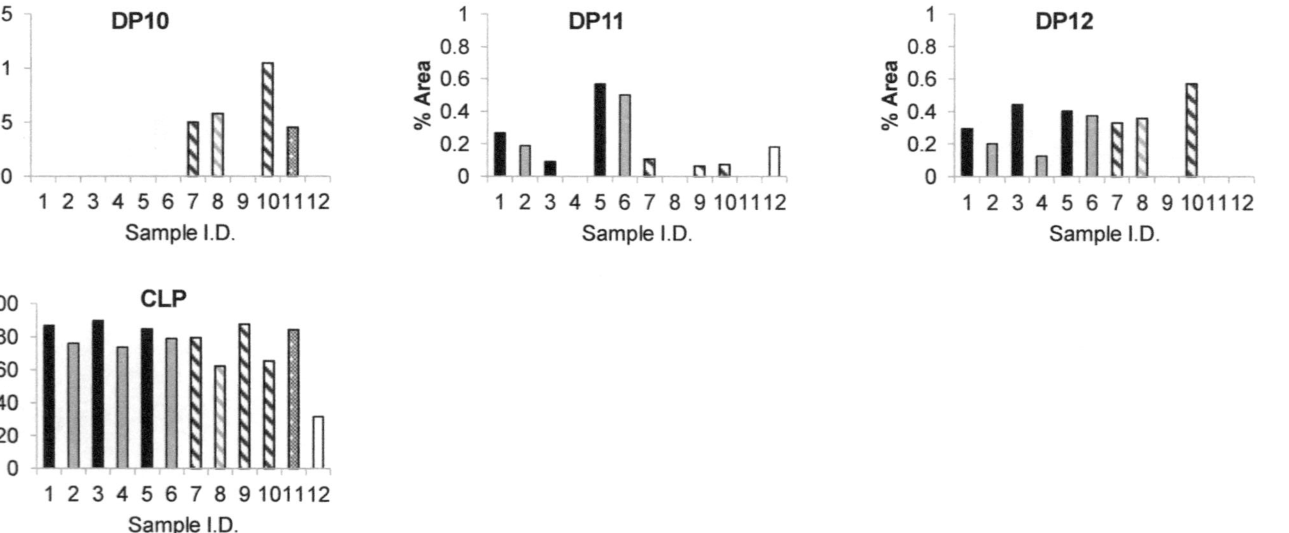


**Figure 3.** Overview of the HPLC-UV sample measurement results: amount of formed DPs 1-12 and CLP (n = 2). The columns are colored and pattered according to the stressing conditions: steel jar (blue), $ZrO_2$ jar (black), oxone 10% m/m (filled), oxone 2% m/m (striped), without stressor (dotted), $KNO_3$ (white, no filling).

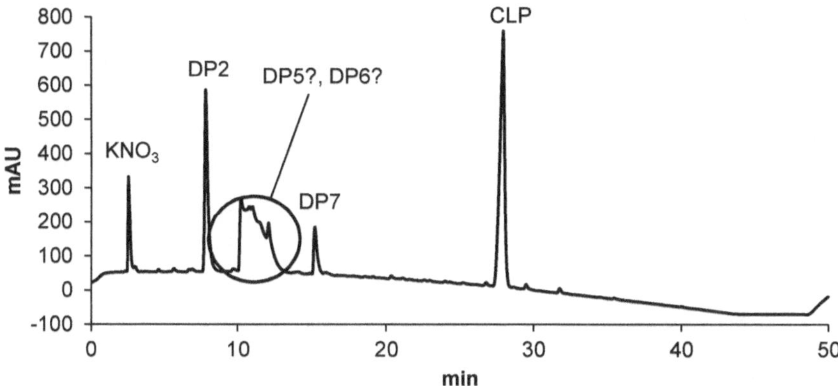



**Figure 4.** Chromatogram of sample 12 (stressed with KNO₃).

## 3.4 Identification of degradation products using MS

7 of the 12 DPs detected by HPLC-UV could be characterized by their mass-to-charge ratios (m/z). Reliable m/z of the remaining DPs could not be determined. Structural elucidation was supported by the respective fragmentation spectra and by comparison with structures already identified in the literature. An overview is shown in Tab. 6. The mass spectra of CLP and its major degradant (DP4, CLP acid) are depicted in Fig. 6 - 9, respectively.

**Table 6.** Overview of the potential CLP degradation products (DPs).

| | Structure | m/z | Chemical formula |
|---|---|---|---|
| DP2 | | 306 | $C_{15}H_{13}NO_2SCl$ |
| DP4 | | 308 | $C_{15}H_{15}NO_2SCl$ |

Degradation profiling of Clopidogrel hydrogen sulfate stressed in the solid state using mechanochemistry under oxidative conditions

| | | | |
|---|---|---|---|
| **DP5** | 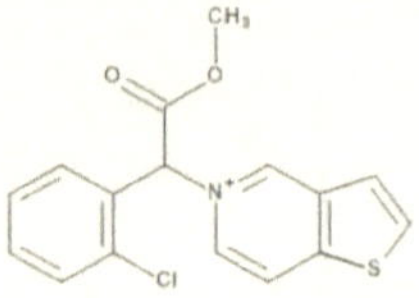 | 318 | $C_{16}H_{13}NO_2SCl$ |
| **DP6** | 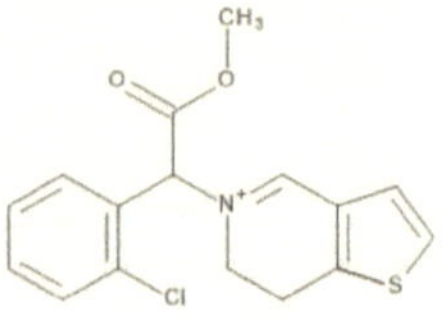 | 320 | $C_{16}H_{15}NO_2SCl$ |
| **DP7** | 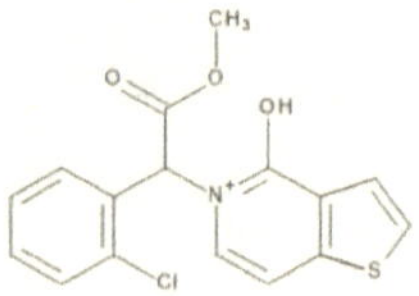 or 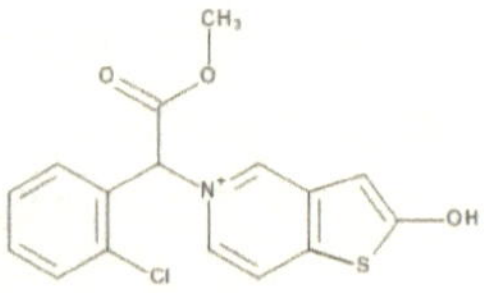 | 334 | $C_{16}H_{13}NO_3SCl$ |
| **DP8** | 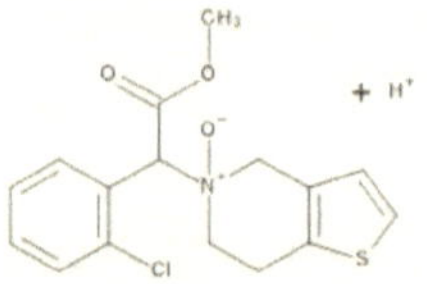 | 338 | $C_{16}H_{17}NO_3SCl$ |
| **DP9** | 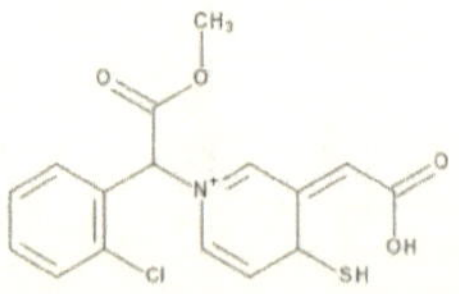 | 352 | $C_{16}H_{15}NO_4SCl$ |

*DP2 (m/z 306)*

The m/z of the main peak and its corresponding fragment was found to be 306 and 138, respectively. The structure of *DP2* was already identified and suggested to be formed by ester hydrolysis and dehydrogenation of CLP under neutral and basic, but not under acidic conditions [16]. Moreover, as shown by this study, it was found to be a major degradation product if $KNO_3$ was applied as oxidizing agent (Fig. 4).

*DP4 (m/z 308)*

*DP4* was the major degradation product in every stressed sample measured. The compound was identified as CLP acid with an m/z of 308 which was confirmed by the fragment pattern including the m/z 198, 169, 152, 141 and 125, which was reported by Raijda et al. [16] (Fig. 5, 7 - 9). CLP acid is specified in the Ph.Eur. and the United States Pharmacopoeia (USP) as impurity A and related compound A, respectively (Tab. 7) [20,23]. It is formed by ester hydrolysis of CLP, which occurs in solution or in solid state under basic, acidic or neutral stress conditions [12-14,16,20,22]. As observed in this study, it is also formed under oxidative conditions in the solid state, especially if high amounts of catalyst and $SiO_2$-oxone-ratios were applied (samples 7 and 8).

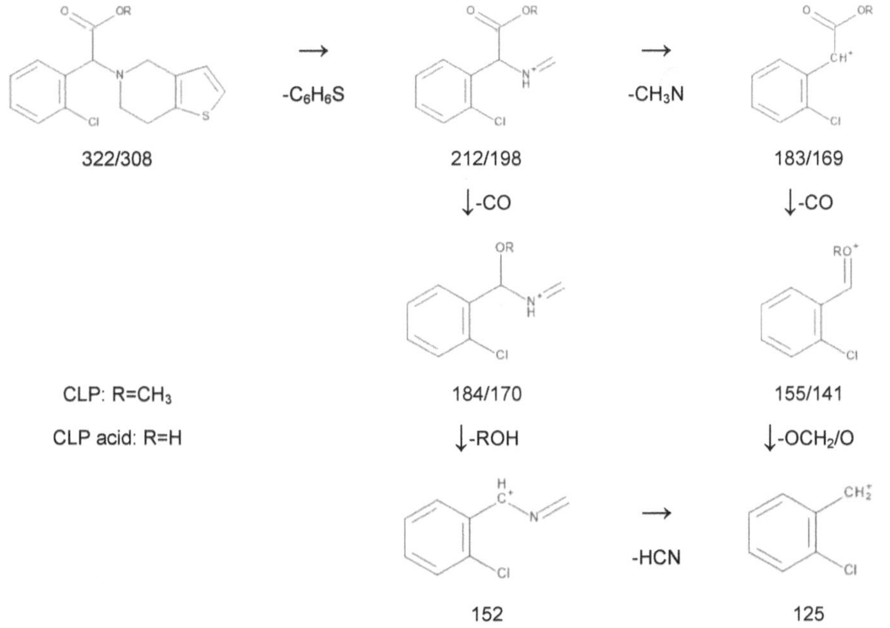

**Figure 5.** Fragmentation profile of CLP and CLP acid supported with the m/z as described by Raijda et al [16].

Degradation profiling of Clopidogrel hydrogen sulfate stressed in the solid state using mechanochemistry under oxidative conditions

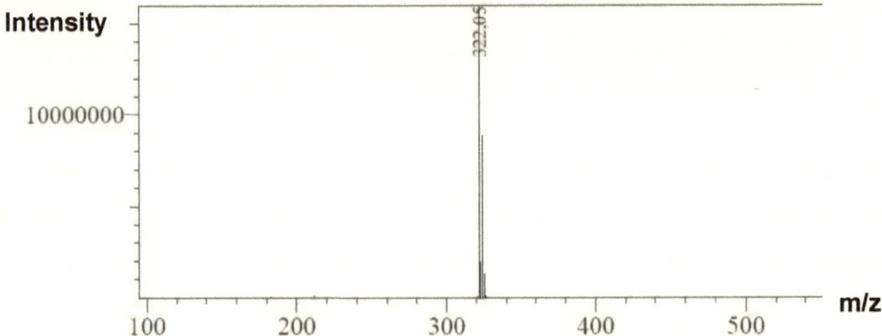

**Figure 6.** Mass spectrum of CLP (M+H)$^+$ = 322.

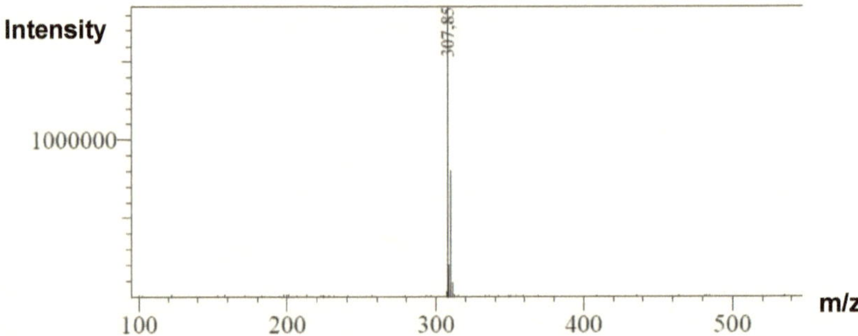

**Figure 7.** Mass spectrum of DP4 (M+H)$^+$ = 308.

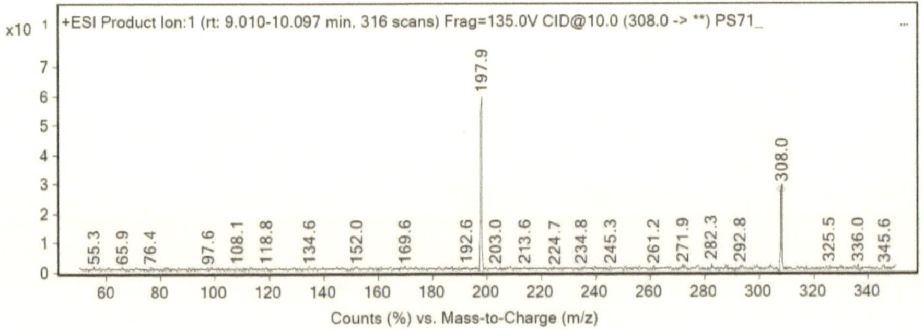

**Figure 8.** Fragmentation spectrum of DP4 (collision energy 10 eV).

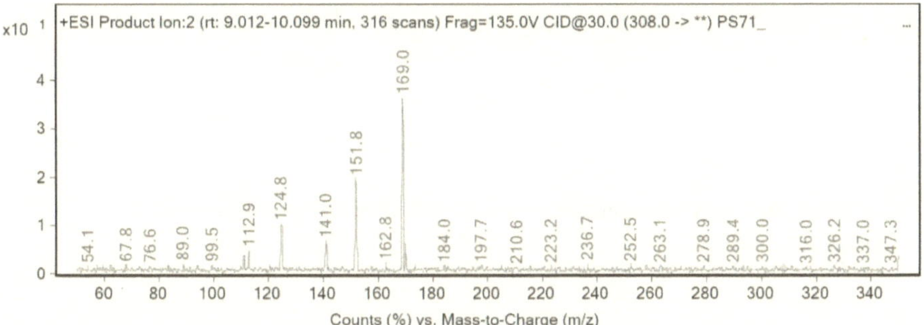


**Figure 9.** Fragmentation spectrum of DP4 (collision energy 30 eV).

*DP5 (m/z 318)*

A compound with m/z 318 was used by Kashay et al. as a reference substance for an LC method development, but its formation under stressing conditions has not been studied [12]. The m/z of 318 is indicative of a dehydrogenation of the CLP drug (m/z 322) under oxidative conditions, resulting in aromatization of the piperidine heterocycle. The m/z of the fragments were 183 and 155, respectively, indicating the precursor substance to be the CLP methylated ester (see Fig. 5). Our study showed that the formation of *DP5* was more intense in steel than in $ZrO_2$ jars, which points to the different reactivities of the jar materials.

*DP6 (m/z 320)*

In the literature, two different decomposition products of CLP with an m/z 320 are reported: the first one results from a dehydrogenation process of the CLP drug, and hence might be a possible precursor of *DP5* [12,17,18]. It was formed by accelerated stability testing of a physical drug-excipient-mixture (incubated at 80 °C for 3 days), and under oxidative conditions ($H_2O_2$ 5% V/V, 60 °C, 3 hours) [18]. As a second option, an m/z of 320 is referred to a dehydrogenated, hydroxylated derivative of CLP-acid (Fig. 10), which is a minor DP of the amorphous form of CLP and formed under neutral conditions [16]. However, an m/z of 155 detected in the fragmentation spectrum of *DP6* indicates a methylated ester as a precursor. Hence, *DP6* rather refers to the structure described by Mohan et al. and Aparna et al. (Tab. 6). Moreover, the UV/Vis spectra of *DP6* and *"related compound D"* [18] were found to be similar. As observed for *DP5*, *DP6* also shows enhanced formation during mechanochemical stressing if steel was selected as ball mill material.

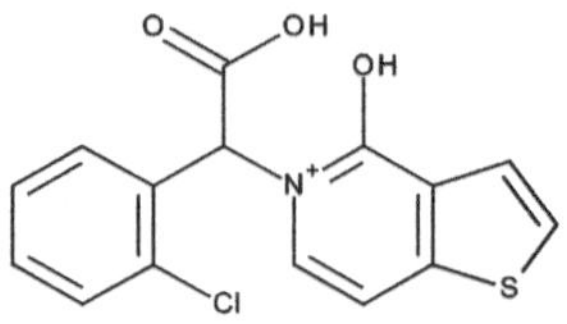

**Figure 10.** Degradation product (m/z 320) of CLP found by Raijda et al [16].

*DP7 (m/z 334)*

The structure with an m/z of 334 has been reported by Raijda et al [16], which is formed as a minor degradation product of amorphous CLP under neutral conditions. It might result from the hydroxylation of *DP5*, the suggested structure is depicted in Table 6. However, the hydroxylation may also take place in position C-15 of the thiophene as it is the case for the activation of CLP *in vivo* [8]. In this study, it was found to be a major degradation product if milled with $KNO_3$.

*DP8 (m/z 338)*

The substance with an m/z of 338 may refer to the CLP *N*-oxide, which was formed under oxidative conditions only as reported by Mashelkar and Renapurkar [14]. Interestingly, the formation of *DP8* was not observed if $KNO_3$ was used as the oxidizing agent.

*DP9 (m/z 352)*

*DP9* showed an m/z of 352, a possible structure is depicted in Tab. 6. It might be the dehydrogenated derivative of the bioactive CLP thiol metabolite (Fig. 1). Forced degradation studies carried out on the CLP drug substance/product have not reported on this DP yet.

All the structures observed in this study are described as CLP decomposition products in the literature, but only *DP6* and *DP8* were identified under oxidative conditions yet. As mentioned above, Buschmann and Handler performed initial tests for degradation profiling of CLP using mechanochemistry [7]. Here, $KMnO_4$ on aluminium oxide was used as a catalyst for the oxidative solid state stress test. Two degradation products were observed, but not further identified; one of them is assumed to be the didehydro CLP, which may correspond to *DP6*. Interestingly, an m/z of 324 (CLP acid *N*-oxide) could not be observed, which was found in [14] under oxidative conditions. The peaks at 1 - 4 min did not give satisfactory results upon m/z analysis. However, as mentioned above, the peaks are not related to the catalyst matrix. According to their retention behavior on the C8 column, the peaks are expected to represent polar compounds, which may apply to the end products of the CLP decomposition process [16]. Further investigations of the broad hump of the unresolved peaks in the chromatogram of sample 12 (Fig. 4) were performed by means of MS. Among others, the m/z 320 (presumably *DP6*), 356, 364 and 413 could be detected. Obviously, neither UV nor MS analysis could confirm the formation of CLP acid when $KNO_3$ was used as the oxidative stressor. The m/z 356 may be assigned to the active metabolite of CLP (Fig. 1), which, however, was not further investigated. No CLP derived compound was described in the literature employing the m/z of 364 and 413. Due to the high m/z compared to other DPs identified, the respective structures might result from unknown oxidation processes, which should be further investigated. Apart from CLP acid, the Ph.Eur. and USP monograph of CLP hydrogen sulfate does not report on any other DP found in this study (Tab. 7).

**Table 7.** Transparency list of the CLP hydrogen sulfate monograph of the Ph.Eur. and the USP [20,23].

| Impurity/related compound | IUPAC description | Structure | M_r |
|---|---|---|---|
| A | (2S)-(2-chlorophenyl)[6,7-dihydrothieno[3,2-c]pyridin-5(4H)-yl]acetic acid | 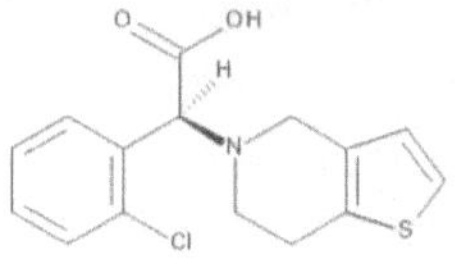 | 307 |
| B | Methyl-(2S)-(2-chlorophenyl)[4,7-dihydrothieno[2,3-c]pyridin-6(5H)-yl]acetate | 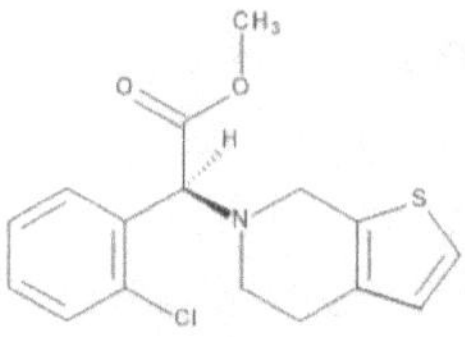 | 321 |
| C | Methyl-(2R)-(2-chlorophenyl)[6,7-dihydrothieno[3,2-c]pyridin-5(4H)-yl]acetate | 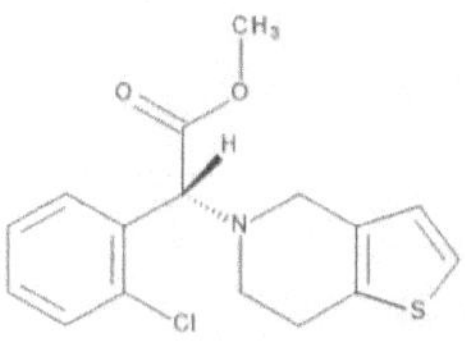 | 321 |

| D<br>(non-specified impurity of the Ph.Eur.) | Methyl-(2*R*)-(2-chlorophenyl)[(2*S*)-(2-chlorophenyl)[6,7-dihydrothieno[3,2-*c*]pyridin-5(4*H*)-yl]acetyloxy]acetate | | 505 |

## 3.5 Estimation of LOD and LOQ of the degradation products

For the estimation of the LOD and LOQ of the DPs, differences in their molar extinction coefficients and molar masses (relative to CLP) were considered by using correction factors.

Several structural changes of the CLP parent compound can occur during stressing, such as hydrogenation and hydroxylation of the thienopyridine moiety or hydrolysis of the methyl ester. This may affect the chromophore of the molecule and lead to shifting absorptions bands in the UV/Vis spectrum, which was considered by normalizing the UV/Vis spectra of all and setting the absorbances at $\lambda = 235$ nm of the DPs in relation to that of CLP. Moreover, the UV/Vis detector response is dependent on the amount of substance to be analyzed, which was considered by applying the ratios of the molar masses of CLP and the DPs. The LODs and LOQs of the DPs were calculated according to section 2.4.3, using the correction factors (reciprocal of the RRF). The estimated LODs and LOQs of the DPs are summarized in Tab. 8.

The LODs and LOQs ranged from 0.23 to 1.74 µg/mL (0.02 - 0.17%) and from 0.76 to 5.80 µg/mL (0.08 - 0.58%), respectively. For *DP8*, LOD and LOQ were not determined, because samples containing *DP8* were only analyzed with the non-optimized, less sensitive HPLC-UV method.

**Table 8.** Estimated LOD and LOQ of the detected degradation products (DPs).
RFF: relative response factor; n.a.: not available.

| DP | RRF | LOD | | LOQ | |
|---|---|---|---|---|---|
| | | (µg/mL) | (%) | (µg/mL) | (%) |
| 1 | 0.503 | 0.57 | 0.06 | 1.92 | 0.19 |
| 2 | 1.061 | 0.37 | 0.04 | 1.24 | 0.12 |
| 3 | 0.576 | 0.78 | 0.08 | 2.60 | 0.26 |
| 4 | 0.859 | 0.60 | 0.06 | 2.00 | 0.20 |
| 5 | 1.039 | 0.70 | 0.07 | 2.34 | 0.23 |
| 6 | 0.519 | 1.74 | 0.17 | 5.80 | 0.58 |
| 7 | 1.505 | 0.23 | 0.02 | 0.76 | 0.08 |
| 8 | n.a. | n.a. | n.a. | n.a. | n.a. |
| 9 | 0.883 | 0.41 | 0.04 | 1.36 | 0.14 |
| 10 | 0.371 | 0.89 | 0.09 | 2.96 | 0.30 |
| 11 | 1.015 | 0.73 | 0.07 | 2.43 | 0.24 |
| 12 | 0.926 | 0.33 | 0.03 | 1.10 | 0.11 |

## 4. Conclusion

In this study, the degradation of CLP under oxidative conditions applying solid state
mechanochemistry was investigated. An already existing MS compatible LC method
was adjusted for the separation of various DPs, which were subsequently
characterized by their UV and mass spectra. Most of the peaks could be assigned to
structures which were obtained from various CLP stressing tests described in the
literature. Many DPs identified in this study were reported to be observed under
acidic or basic, but not under oxidative conditions. The amount of degradation and its
profile was influenced by the jar material, milling frequency, and the type of catalyst
used. The study supports the findings by Buschmann and Handler [7] and clearly
demonstrates that mechanochemistry is a valuable alternative for stress tests carried
out in the liquid state.

# 5. References

[1] International Council for Harmonization, Guideline Q1A(R2): *Stability Testing Of New Drug Substances and Products* 2003.

[2] T. Rawat, I.P. Pandey, Forced degradation studies for Drug Substances and Drug Products-Scientific and Regulatory Considerations. J. Pharm. Sci. Res. 2015, 7, 238-241.

[3] International Council for Harmonization, Guideline Q1B: *Stability Testing: Photostability Testing of New Drug Substances and Products* 1996.

[4] S.L. James, P. Collier, I. Parkin, G. Hyett, D. Braga, L. Maini, B. Jones, T. Friščić, C. Bolm, A. Krebs, J. Mack, D.C. Waddell, W.C. Shearouse, G. Orpen, C. Adams, J.W. Steed, K.D.M. Harris, Mechanochemistry: opportunities for new and cleaner synthesis. Chem. Soc. Rev. 2012, 41, 413-447.

[5] J.G. Hernández, C. Bolm, Altering product selectivity by mechanochemistry. J. Org. Chem. 2017, 82, 4007-4019.

[6] T. Friščić, C. Mottillo, H.M. Titi, Mechanochemistry for synthesis. Angew. Chem. Int. Ed. 2020, 59, 1018-1029.

[7] H.H. Buschmann, N. Handler, Mechanochemical process in a Solid State Reaction, WIPO (PCT) world patent WO 2018/096066 A1, 2018 May 31.

[8] Kommentar zum Europäischen Arzneibuch, Monographie 7.1/2531 – Clopidogrelhydrogensulfat. 52. Aktualisierungslieferung, Wissenschaftliche Verlagsgesellschaft Stuttgart, Stuttgart, 2015.

[9] P.J. Sharis, C.P. Cannon, J. Loscalzo, The Antiplatelet Effects of Ticlopidine and Clopidogrel. Ann. Intern. Med. 1998, 129, 394-405.

[10] J.M. Herbert, D. Frehel, E. Vallee, G. Kieffer, D. Gouy, Y. Berger, J. Necciari, G. Defreyn, J.P. Maffrand, Clopidogrel, A Novel Antiplatelet and Antithrombotic Agent. Cardiovasc. Drug Rev. 1993, 11, 180-198.

[11] P. Savi, J.M. Pereillo, M.F. Uzabiaga, J. Combalbert, C. Picard, J.P. Maffrand, M. Pascal, J.M. Herbert, Identification and Biological Activity of the Active Metabolite of Clopidogrel. Thromb. Haemost. 2000, 84, 891-896.

[12] G. Kahsay, A. Van Schepdael, E. Adams, Development and validation of a liquid chromatographic method for purity control of clopidogrel–acetylsalicylic acid in combined oral dosage forms. J. Pharm. Biomed. Anal 2012, 61, 271-276.

[13] P.R. Deshmukh, V.L. Gaikwad, P.K. Tamane, K.R. Mahadik, R.N. Purohit, Development of stability-indicating HPLC method and accelerated stability studies for osmotic and pulsatile tablet formulations of Clopidogrel Bisulfate. J. Pharm. Biomed. Anal. 2019, 165, 346-356.

[14] U.C. Mashelkar, S.D. Renapurkar, A LCMS compatible stability-indicating HPLC assay method for clopidogrel bisulphate, Int. J. Chem. Tech. Res. 2010, 2, 822-829.

[15] A. Mitakos, I. Panderi, A validated LC method for the determination of clopidogrel in pharmaceutical preparations, J. Pharm. Biomed. Anal. 2002, 28, 431-438.

[16] D.K. Raijada, B. Prasad, A. Paudel, R.P. Shah, S. Singh, Characterization of degradation products of amorphous and polymorphic forms of clopidogrel bisulfate under solid state stress conditions, J. Pharm. Biomed. Anal., 2010, 52, 332-344.

[17] P. Aparna, S.V. Rao, K.M. Thomas, K. Mukkanti, K. Deo, Non chiral High Performance Liquid Chromatography method for monitoring unknown impurities generated during stability of clopidogrel tablets. Der Pharma Chem. 2010, 2, 244-252.

[18] A. Mohan, M. Hariharan, E. Vikraman, G. Subbaiah, B.R. Venkataraman, D. Saravanan, Identification and characterization of a principal oxidation impurity in clopidogrel drug substance and drug product. J. Pharm. Biomed. Anal. 2008, 47, 183-189.

[19] M. Takahashi, H. Pang, K. Kawabata, N.A. Farid, A. Kurihara, Quantitative determination of clopidogrel active metabolite in human plasma by LC-MS/MS. J. Pharm. Biomed. Anal. 2008, 48, 1219-1224.

[20] EDQM, Strasbourg, France. Monograph No. 01/2017:2531 corrected 10.0 –
Clopidogrel hydrogen sulfate. European Pharmacopoeia Online 10.4, 2020.

[21] International Council for Harmonization, Guideline Q2(R1): *Validation of
Analytical Procedures: Text and Methodology* 1996.

[22] EDQM, Strasbourg, France. Chapter 2.2.46 – Chromatographic Separation
Techniques. European Pharmacopoeia Online 10.4, 2020.

[23] Clopidogrel bisulfate official monograph, United States Pharmacopeia, 42 ed.,
The United States Pharmacopeial Convention, Rockville, MD, 2020.

# 4. Final Discussion

The objective of this book was to elaborate appropriate methods for the quality control of APIs and excipients. In the projects, different techniques were employed to address the specific analytical problem: NMR spectroscopy was used for the evaluation of MOAH in paraffins and the impurity profiling of L-ascorbic acid-2-phosphate (A2PMg). The isomerization of Ibu and decomposition of Clopidogrel, induced by solid-state mechanochemistry, were studied by establishing appropriate CE and HPLC methods with suitable detection, respectively.

## 4.1 Evaluation of MOAH in paraffins

Paraffins are mineral oil based mixtures of highly alkylated compounds (MOH), which comprise saturated (MOSH) and aromatic hydrocarbons (MOAH). If paraffins are intended for pharmaceutical use, residues of potentially carcinogenic polycyclic aromatic compounds (PAH) have to be removed during refining, which is tested for in the compendial monographs. This test is not applicable to further characterize the paraffins because it only limits the amount of PAH, whereas the monocyclic aromatic hydrocarbons (MAH) and the MOSH are disregarded. However, knowledge about those compounds may be crucial to e.g. provide a better tracking of the refinement process, study the composition of the paraffins and thus implement a "fingerprint" of a paraffin sample. Several methods have been reported for the analysis of MOSH and MOAH [1]. The gold standard is based on LC-GC-FID, which, however, is a conventional method and requires exact operating, elaborate sample preparation, and comprehensive know-how for interpretation of results.

A method based on $^1$H NMR spectroscopy was developed as a straightforward alternative for the evaluation of MOAH in paraffins. Major advantages were the selective detection of MOSH and MOAH, rapid and easy sample preparation, and simple interpretation of results. The amount of MOAH was evaluated by relating the integral of the MOAH to that of the MOSH protons. The MOAH/MOSH ratio was successfully applied to a highly diverse paraffin sample pool to examine the extent of refining. Synthetic and liquid paraffins showed the lowest amount of MOAH, which increased for soft paraffins and was highest for paraffins for technical use and paraffin refining intermediates.

The $^1$H NMR measurement results were supported by those from the UV spectroscopic purity test of paraffins according to DAB 8. The UV absorbances are indicative of the amount of MAOH, and by selecting the appropriate measuring wavelength, a rough distinction can be made between MAH and PAH [2]. Therefore, the $^1$H NMR and UV spectroscopic methods were compared by correlating the absorbances (A) at the various wavelengths with the MOAH/MOSH ratios of the paraffin samples. This resulted in an approximating linear relationship; highest correlations were found for PAH/MOSH vs. A (295 nm) ($R^2 = 0.977$) and lowest for MAH/MOSH vs. A (295 nm) ($R^2 = 0.626$). For appropriate interpretation of results, overlapping resonances or absorption bands of the MOAH have to be considered, as well as the fact that the MOAH/MOSH ratio depends on the extent of alkylation of the aromatic core.

Finally, PCA was used as an explorative, unsupervised chemometric tool to identify groups within the paraffin samples. A distinction could be made according to the consistency of the paraffins (soft, liquid, and solid), and natural liquid paraffins could be separated from the artificially produced. The main variance of the paraffins was due to the large MOSH integral, whereas the MOAH did not contribute to any grouping within the paraffin samples.

## 4.2 Impurity profiling of L-ascorbic acid-2-phosphate magnesium

NMR spectroscopy is an excellent tool for structural elucidation and is therefore not only used in organic synthesis, but also in quality control of APIs and excipients [3]. The most common nuclei detected by NMR spectroscopy are $^1$H and $^{13}$C, but the study of other nuclei, such as $^{15}$N, $^{19}$F and $^{31}$P, can be helpful in some cases. A variety of one- and multidimensional NMR techniques is available to obtain as much structural information as possible about the molecule of interest [4].

One- and two-dimensional $^1$H, $^{13}$C and $^{31}$P NMR spectroscopy has been applied to examine the impurity profile of A2PMg and to support previous findings obtained by MS studies [5]. Therefore, crude A2PMg and fractions thereof collected from preparative HPLC were analyzed. Several phosphorylated and ethylated impurities could be detected, which were likely to be formed during synthesis of A2PMg. Overall, the structures of four impurities were identified (Tab. 1). The structure of ascorbic acid 2-phosphate-ethylester (Imp. d) suggested by MS could be confirmed.

**Table 1.** Impurities of A2PMg identified with NMR spectroscopy.

| Ascorbic acid 2-phosphate-ethyl ester (Imp. d) | Ascorbic acid 3,5-diphosphate (Imp. i) | Ascorbic acid 5-phosphate (Imp. h) | Ethanol |
| --- | --- | --- | --- |

## 4.3 Degradation of mechanochemically stressed APIs

Forced degradation studies (stress tests) are performed on drug substances and products as part of the stability-indicating studies described by the ICH guideline Q1A(R2) to establish the degradation profile of a drug [6]. Common stress tests are carried out in the liquid state under basic, acidic, or oxidizing conditions. As an alternative, solid-state mechanochemistry can be applied, where the substance to be examined is stressed in the solid state under the influence of mechanical energy, which is provided by e.g. ball mills [7]. The mechanical energy input can be varied by adjusting the milling time and speed for instance. Acidic, basic or oxidizing environment can be generated by adding appropriate (solid) stressors such as NaOH platelets or oxone. The applicability of solid-state mechanochemistry for forced degradation studies was investigated on two APIs, including Dexibuprofen (*S*-Ibu) and Clopidogrel (CLP).

For the examination of the isomerization of *S*-Ibu in the solid-state, an enantioselective CE method was developed and validated according to ICH Q2(R1). It was shown that the addition of divalent cations to the running buffer, such as $Mg^{2+}$ and $Zn^{2+}$ salts, significantly improved resolution of the Ibu isomers. Several rinsing procedures between consecutive runs were tested to obtain reproducible migration times. The final method was applied on a series of variously stressed *S*-Ibu samples. *S*-Ibu was found to isomerize under basic conditions at high milling time and speed, but to a very low extent of a few percent. Hence, *S*-Ibu is expected to be stereochemically stable under common storage conditions.

The degradation profile of solid-state stressed CLP was studied using HPLC-UV and HPLC-MS/(MS). The HPLC method used for the compendial test on related substances of CLP was considered inappropriate, because it is not compatible with MS detection. Therefore, a stability-indicating HPLC method suitable for MS coupling was selected from the literature and adjusted to achieve sufficient separation of the degradation products. The method was applied to CLP samples, which were stressed using varying amounts of oxone and $KNO_3$ as oxidizing agents, and two different jar/ball materials. Among the various formed degradation products, 7 were structurally elucidated, which were already described in literature. Since the majority of the degradation products were not commercially available, the corresponding quantification limits were established by estimating the relative response factors, which were obtained from the normalized UV/Vis spectra.

# References


[1] S. Weber, K. Schrag, G. Mildau, T. Kuballa, S.G. Walch, D.W. Lachenmeier, Analytical Methods for the Determination of Mineral Oil Saturated Hydrocarbons (MOSH) and Mineral Oil Aromatic Hydrocarbons (MOAH) – A Short Review. Anal. Chem. Insights 2018, 13, 1-16.

[2] H. Böhme, W. Hühnermann, Probleme des Arzneibuches. Zur Untersuchung der Mineralölprodukte im Deutschen Arzneibuch, 7. Ausgabe. Arch. Pharm. 1966, 299, 368-380.

[3] U. Holzgrabe, I. Wawer, B. Diehl (Eds.), NMR Spectroscopy in Pharmaceutical Analysis, 1st ed., Elsevier, Oxford, UK, 2008.

[4] O. Zerbe, S. Jurt, Applied NMR Spectroscopy for Chemists and Life Scientists. Wiley-VCH, Weinheim, 2014.

[5] X. Xu, J. Urlaub, M. Woźniczka, E. Wynendaele, K. Herman, C. Schollmayer, B. Diehl, S. Van Calenbergh, U. Holzgrabe, B. De Spiegeleer, Zwitterionic-hydrophilic interaction liquid chromatography for L-ascorbic acid 2-phosphate magnesium, a raw material in cell therapy. J. Pharm. Biomed. Anal. 2019, 165, 338-345.

[6] International Council for Harmonization, Guideline Q1A(R2): Stability Testing Of New Drug Substances and Products 2003.

[7] H.H. Buschmann, N. Handler, Mechanochemical process in a Solid State Reaction, WIPO (PCT) world patent WO 2018/096066 A1, 2018 May 31.

# 5. Summary

For the quality assurance of substances for pharmaceutical use, a variety of analytical techniques are available to address specific analytical problems. In this field of application, liquid chromatography (LC) stands out as the gold standard in the pharmaceutical industry. Various detectors can be employed, which are e.g. based on UV/Vis spectroscopy for the examination of molecules with a chromophore, or mass spectrometry (MS) for structural elucidation of analytes. For the separation of enantiomers, the use of capillary electrophoresis (CE) may be more favorable due to the high separation efficiency and easy-to-use and comparatively inexpensive chiral selectors, in contrast to chiral columns for LC, which are usually very expensive and limited to a restricted number of analytes. For structure elucidation in impurity profiling, one- and multidimensional $^1$H NMR spectroscopy is a valuable tool as long as the analyte molecule has got nuclei that can be detected, which applies for the magnitude of organic pharmaceutical substances.

For the evaluation of the amount of mineral oil aromatic hydrocarbons (MOAH) in various paraffin samples from different suppliers, a straightforward method based on $^1$H NMR spectroscopy was elaborated. The MOAH/MOSH ratio was used to indicate the amount of MOAH of paraffins and to evaluate the extent of refining. In addition, a representative paraffin sample was measured without sample solvent at high temperatures (about 340 K) to avoid the interfering residual solvent signals in the spectral regions of interest. The results of both methods were in good accordance.

Moreover, the $^1$H NMR results were complemented with the UV measurements from the purity testing of paraffins according to the DAB 8. Correlations of the NMR and UV spectroscopic data indicated a linear relationship of both methods for the determination of MOAH in paraffins.

Finally, the $^1$H NMR data was evaluated by principal component analysis (PCA) to explore differences within the paraffin samples and the spectral regions in the $^1$H NMR spectrum which are responsible for the formation of groups. It could be found that most variation is due to the MOSH of the paraffins. The PCA model was capable of differentiating between soft, liquid and solid paraffins on the one hand and between natural and synthetic liquid paraffins on the other hand.

The impurity profiling of L-ascorbic acid 2-phosphate magnesium (A2PMg) was performed by means of one- and two-dimensional NMR spectroscopy. Several ethylated impurities could be detected, which were likely to be formed during synthesis of A2PMg. The structures of two of the ethylated impurities were identified as ascorbic acid 2-phosphate ethyl ester and ethanol, (residual solvent from synthesis). NMR spectroscopic studies of the fractions obtained from preparative HPLC of A2PMg revealed two additional impurities, which were identified as phosphorylated derivatives of ascorbic acid, ascorbic acid 3,5-phosphate and ascorbic acid 5-phosphate.

Solid state mechanochemistry as an alternative approach for stress testing was applied on the drug substances $S$-Ibuprofen (Ibu) and Clopidogrel (CLP) using a ball mill, in order to study their degradation profile:

First, the isomerization of $S$-Ibu was investigated, which was stressed in the solid state applying several milling frequencies and durations under basic, acidic and neutral conditions. For the separation of Ibu enantiomers, a chiral CE method was developed and validated according to ICH Q2(R1). It was found that $S$-Ibu is overall very stable to isomerization; it shows minor conversion into the $R$-enantiomer under basic environment applying long milling times and high frequencies.

Last, the degradation profile of clopidogrel hydrogen sulfate (CLP) was investigated, which was stressed in the solid state under various oxidative conditions. An already existing HPLC-UV method was adjusted to sufficiently separate the degradation products, which were characterized by means of UV and MS/(MS) detection. Most of the degradation products identified were already reported to result from conventional CLP stress tests. The degradation profile of CLP was mainly influenced by the material of the milling jar and the type of catalyst used.

# 6. Zusammenfassung

Für die Qualitätssicherung von Arznei- und Hilfsstoffen steht eine Vielzahl von analytischen Techniken für spezifische analytische Fragestellungen zur Verfügung. In der pharmazeutischen Industrie hat sich dabei die Flüssigkeitschromatographie als Goldstandard etabliert. Es können verschiedene Detektoren eingesetzt werden, die z. B. auf UV/Vis-Spektroskopie zur Untersuchung von Molekülen mit einem Chromophor oder auf Massenspektrometrie zur Strukturaufklärung von Analyten basieren. Für die Trennung von Enantiomeren kann die Verwendung von Kapillarelektrophorese aufgrund der hohen Trenneffizienz und der einfach zu handhabenden und vergleichsweise preiswerten chiralen Selektoren gegenüber chiralen Säulen in der Flüssigchromatographie bevorzugt sein, die in der Regel sehr teuer und auf eine begrenzte Anzahl von Analyten beschränkt sind. Für die Strukturaufklärung im Rahmen der Erstellung von Verunreinigungsprofilen ist die ein- und mehrdimensionale $^1$H-NMR-Spektroskopie eine sehr wertvolle Methode, solange das Analytmolekül Kerne besitzt, die der NMR-Spektroskopie zugänglich sind, was für den Großteil der organischen Arznei- und Hilfsstoffe zutrifft.

Um die Menge an „mineral oil aromatic hydrocarbons (MOAH)" in verschiedenen Paraffinproben von unterschiedlichen Herstellern zu bestimmen, wurde eine einfache $^1$H-NMR-Spektroskopie-Methode erarbeitet. Das Verhältnis von MOAH zu „mineral oil saturated hydrocarbons (MOSH)" wurde dazu verwendet, um die Menge der MOAH in Paraffinen zu bestimmen und ihren Raffinationsgrad zu beurteilen. Zusätzlich wurde eine repräsentative Paraffinprobe ohne Probenlösungsmittel bei hohen Temperaturen (ca. 340 K) vermessen, um die interferierenden Restlösemittel-Signale in den relevanten Spektralbereichen zu vermeiden. Die Ergebnisse beider Methoden stimmten gut überein.

Weiterhin wurden die $^1$H-NMR-Ergebnisse durch die UV-Messungen aus der Reinheitsprüfung von Paraffinen gemäß DAB 8 ergänzt. Korrelationen der NMR- und UV-spektroskopischen Daten wiesen auf eine lineare Beziehung beider Methoden für die Bestimmung der MOAH in Paraffinen hin.

Schließlich wurden die $^1$H-NMR-spektroskopischen Daten mittels Hauptkomponentenanalyse ausgewertet, um Unterschiede innerhalb der Paraffinproben und die für die Gruppenbildung verantwortlichen Spektralbereiche im

$^1$H-NMR-Spektrum zu ermitteln. Es konnte festgestellt werden, dass der Hauptanteil der Varianz auf die MOSH zurückzuführen ist. Das PCA-Modell war dazu in der Lage, zwischen weichen, flüssigen und festen Paraffinen einerseits und zwischen natürlichen und synthetischen flüssigen Paraffinen andererseits zu unterscheiden.

Das Verunreinigungsprofil von L-Ascorbinsäure-2-phosphat-Magnesium (A2PMg) wurde mittels ein- und zweidimensionaler NMR-Spektroskopie untersucht. Es konnten mehrere ethylierte Verunreinigungen nachgewiesen werden, die vermutlich während des Syntheseprozesses von A2PMg gebildet wurden. Die Strukturen von zwei der ethylierten Verunreinigungen wurden als Ascorbinsäure-2-phosphat-ethylester und Ethanol (Restlösungsmittel aus der Synthese) identifiziert. NMR-spektroskopische Untersuchungen der aus der präparativen HPLC von A2PMg erhaltenen Fraktionen ergab zwei weitere Verunreinigungen, die als phosphorylierte Derivate von Ascorbinsäure, Ascorbinsäure-3,5-phosphat und Ascorbinsäure-5-phosphat, identifiziert wurden.

Die Festkörper-Mechanochemie als alternativer Ansatz für Stresstests wurde auf die Arzneistoffe S-Ibuprofen und Clopidogrel unter Einsatz einer Kugelmühle angewandt, um deren Abbauprofil zu analysieren:

Zunächst wurde die Isomerisierung von S-Ibuprofen (Ibu) untersucht, das im festen Zustand unter Anwendung verschiedener Mahlfrequenzen und -dauern unter basischen, sauren und neutralen Bedingungen gestresst wurde. Für die Trennung der Ibu-Enantiomere wurde eine chirale Kapillarelektrophorese-Methode entwickelt und gemäß ICH Q2(R1) Leitlinie validiert. Es wurde festgestellt, dass S-Ibu insgesamt sehr stabil gegenüber Isomerisierung ist, jedoch unter basischen Bedingungen und hohen Mahldauern und -frequenzen eine geringe Umwandlung in das R-Enantiomer zeigt.

Zuletzt wurde das Abbauprofil von Clopidogrelhydrogensulfat (CLP) untersucht, das im festen Zustand unter oxidativen Bedingungen gestresst wurde. Eine bereits bestehende HPLC-UV Methode wurde optimiert, um die Abbauprodukte ausreichend zu trennen und anschließend mittels UV- und MS/(MS)-Detektion zu charakterisieren. Die meisten der identifizierten Abbauprodukte waren bereits aus konventionellen CLP-Stresstests bekannt. Das Abbauprofil von CLP wurde hauptsächlich durch das Material der Kugelmühle und den Typ des verwendeten Katalysators beeinflusst.

# 7. Appendix

## 7.1  List of Publications

### Research papers

- <u>Urlaub, J.</u>; Norwig, J.; Schollmayer, C.; Holzgrabe, U. *$^1$H NMR analytical characterization of mineral oil hydrocarbons (PARAFFINS) for pharmaceutical use,* J. Pharm. Biomed. Anal. **2019**, 169, 41-48.

- <u>Urlaub, J.</u>; Norwig, J.; Schollmayer, C.; Holzgrabe, U. *Reply to "Requirements for accurate $^1$H NMR quantification of mineral oil hydrocarbons (paraffins) for pharmaceutical or cosmetic use",* J. Pharm. Biomed. Anal. **2019**, 171, 235-237.

- <u>Urlaub, J.</u>; Kaiser, R. P.; Scherf-Clavel, O.; Bolm, C.; Holzgrabe, U. *Investigation of isomerization of dexibuprofen in a ball mill using chiral capillary electrophoresis.* Electrophoresis **2021**, 0, 1-10.

- Xu, X.; <u>Urlaub. J.</u>; Woźniczka, M.; Wynendaele, E.; Herman, K.; Schollmayer, C.; Diehl, B.; Van Calenbergh, S.; Holzgrabe, U.; De Spiegeleer, B. *Zwitterionic-hydrophilic interaction liquid chromatography for L-ascorbic acid 2-phosphate magnesium, a raw material in cell therapy,* J. Pharm. Biomed. Anal. **2019**, 165, 338-345.

## 7.2 Documentation of Authorship

This section contains a list of the individual contribution for each author to the publications reprinted in this book. Unpublished manuscripts are handled accordingly.

| P1 | Urlaub, J.; Norwig, J.; Schollmayer, C.; Holzgrabe, U. [1]H NMR analytical characterization of mineral oil hydrocarbons (PARAFFINS) for pharmaceutical use. J. Pharm. Biomed. Anal. **2019**, 169, 41-48. | | | | |
|---|---|---|---|---|---|
| **Author** | | **1** | **2** | **3** | **4** |
| Study design | | X | X | | X |
| Experimental work: NMR | | X | | X | |
| Data analysis and interpretation | | X | | | |
| Manuscript planning | | X | | | X |
| Manuscript writing | | X | X | | |
| Correction of manuscript | | X | X | X | X |
| Supervision of Jonas Urlaub | | | | | X |

| P2 | Urlaub, J.; Norwig, J.; Schollmayer, C.; Holzgrabe, U. Reply to „Requirements for accurate [1]H NMR quantification of mineral oil hydrocarbons (paraffins) for pharmaceutical or cosmetic use". J. Pharm. Biomed. Anal. **2019**, 171, 235-237. | | | | |
|---|---|---|---|---|---|
| **Author** | | **1** | **2** | **3** | **4** |
| Manuscript planning | | X | | | X |
| Manuscript writing | | X | X | | X |
| Correction of manuscript | | X | X | X | X |
| Supervision of Jonas Urlaub | | | | | X |

| P3 | **Urlaub, J.; Kaiser, R. P.; Scherf-Clavel, O.; Bolm, C.; Holzgrabe, U.** Investigation of isomerization of dexibuprofen in a ball mill using chiral capillary electrophoresis. Electrophoresis **2021**, 0, 1-10. | | | | | |
|---|---|---|---|---|---|---|
| **Author** | | **1** | **2** | **3** | **4** | **5** |
| Study design | | x | x | x | x | x |
| Experimental work: Sample stressing | | | x | | | |
| Experimental work: CE | | x | | | | |
| Data analysis and interpretation | | x | | | | |
| Manuscript planning | | x | | | | x |
| Manuscript writing | | x | x | | | |
| Correction of manuscript | | x | x | x | x | x |
| Supervision of Jonas Urlaub | | | | | | x |

**Erklärung zu den Eigenanteilen des Doktoranden an Publikationen und Zweitpublikationsrechten bei einer teilkumulativen book.**

Für alle in dieser teilkumulativen book verwendeten Manuskripte liegen die notwendigen Genehmigungen der Verlage („reprint permission‘) für die Zweitpublikation vor, außer das betreffende Kapitel ist nicht publiziert. Dieser Umstand wird einerseits durch die genaue Angabe der Literaturstelle der Erstpublikation auf der ersten Seite des betreffenden Kapitels deutlich gemacht oder die bisherige Nichtveröffentlichung durch den Vermerk „unpublished" oder „nicht veröffentlicht" gekennzeichnet.

Die Mitautoren*innen der in dieser teilkumulativen book verwendeten Manuskripte sind sowohl über die Nutzung als auch über die oben angegebenen Eigenanteile informiert.

Die Beiträge der Mitautoren*innen an den Publikationen sind in den vorausgehenden Tabellen aufgeführt.


Prof. Dr. Ulrike Holzgrabe ______________________        ______________________

                             Ort, Datum                    Unterschrift


Jonas Urlaub         ______________________        ______________________

                             Ort, Datum                    Unterschrift

## 7.3  Conference Contributions

- <u>Urlaub, J.</u>; Schollmayer, C.; Norwig, J.; Diehl, B.; Holzgrabe, U. *Analysis of Mineral Oil Hydrocarbons for Pharmaceutical purposes using $^1H$ NMR spectroscopy.* DPhG Annual meeting, **2018**, Hamburg.

- Urlaub, J. *NMR-Spektroskopische Untersuchungen von Paraffinen und Vaseline,* in: Mineralöl im Fokus des gesundheitlichen Verbraucherschutzes, 17. BfR-Forum Verbraucherschutz, **2017**, Berlin.

## 7.4  List of Abbreviations

| | |
|---|---|
| A2P | L-ascorbic acid 2-phosphate |
| A2PMg | L-ascorbic acid 2-phosphate magnesium |
| ADP | adenosine diphosphate |
| API | active pharmaceutical ingredient |
| AsA | L-ascorbic acid |
| BfArM | Bundesinstitut für Arzneimittel und Medizinprodukte (Federal Institute of Drugs and Medical Devices) |
| BGE | background electrolyte |
| CAD | charged aerosol detector |
| CCQM | committee for chemical measurements |
| CD | cyclodextrin |
| CDR | chiral derivatizing reagent |
| CE | capillary electrophoresis |
| CF | correction factor |
| CGE | capillary gel electrophoresis |
| CLP | clopidogrel |
| CMPA | chiral mobile phase additive |
| CS | chiral selector |
| CSA | chiral solvating agent |
| CSP | chiral stationary phase |
| DAD | diode array detector |
| DNA | desoxyribonucleic acid |
| DP | degradation product |
| DS | dummy scan |

| | |
|---|---|
| EDQM | European Directorate for the Quality of Medicines & Healthcare |
| EOF | electroosmotic flow |
| ERETIC | electronic reference to access *in vivo* concentrations |
| FA | formic acid |
| FDA | Food and Drug Administration |
| FID | flame ionization detection |
| FRC | functional related characteristics |
| GC | gas chromatography |
| HCA | hierarchical cluster analysis |
| HILIC | hydrophilic interaction liquid chromatography |
| HPLC | high performance liquid chromatography |
| Ibu | ibuprofen |
| ICH | International Conference on Harmonization of Technical Requirements for Registration of Pharmaceuticals for Human Use |
| Imp | impurity |
| IP | ion pairing |
| IR | infrared |
| LC | liquid chromatography |
| LOD | limit of detection |
| LOQ | limit of quantification |
| LSR | lanthanide shift reagent |
| MAH | monocyclic aromatic hydrocarbons |
| MEKC | micellar electrokinetic chromatography |
| MOAH | mineral oil aromatic hydrocarbons |
| MOH | mineral oil hydrocarbons |
| MOSH | mineral oil saturated hydrocarbons |

| | |
|---|---|
| MS | mass spectrometry |
| MTPA | α-methoxy-α-(trifluoromethyl)phenylacetic acid |
| m/z | mass-to-charge ratio |
| NDEA | *N*-nitrosodiethylamine |
| NDMA | *N*-nitrosodimethylamine |
| NIR | near infrared |
| NMR | nuclear magnetic resonance |
| NS | number of scans |
| OSCS | oversulfated chondroitin sulfate |
| PAH | polycyclic aromatic hydrocarbons |
| PAT | process analytical technology |
| PCA | principal component analysis |
| PCR | principal component regression |
| Ph.Eur. | European Pharmacopoeia |
| PLS | partial least square |
| ppm | parts per million |
| PULCON | pulse length based concentration determination |
| PVDF | polyvinylidene fluoride |
| qNMR | quantitative nuclear magnetic resonance |
| $R^2$ | coefficient of determination |
| RG | receiver gain |
| ROS | reactive oxidative species |
| RP | reversed phase |
| rpm | rounds per minute |
| RRF | relative response factor |

## List of Abbreviations

---

| | |
|---|---|
| SDS | sodium dodecyl sulfate |
| SIMCA | soft independent modelling of class analogy |
| S/N ratio | signal-to-noise ratio |
| SW | spectral width |
| TD | time domain |
| TFA | trifluoroacetic acid |
| TIC | total ion chromatogram |
| TM-$\beta$-CD | 2,3,6-tri-$O$-methyl-$\beta$-cyclodextrin |
| TMS | tetramethylsilane |
| TSP | 3-(trimethylsilyl)propionic-2,2,3,3-$d_4$ acid |
| USP | United States Pharmacopoeia |
| UV | ultra violet |
| UV/Vis | ultra violet/visible |

## 7.5 Supplementary paper: Zwitterionic-hydrophilic interaction liquid chromatography for L-ascorbic acid 2-phosphate magnesium, a raw material in cell therapy

Xiaolong Xu, <u>Jonas Urlaub</u>[*], Magdalena Woźniczka, Evelien Wynendaele, Karen Herman, Curd Schollmayer, Bernd Diehl, Serge Van Calenbergh, Ulrike Holzgrabe, Bart De Spiegeleer

Reprinted with permission from J. Pharm. Biomed. Anal. 2019, 165, 338-345.

Copyright (2019) Wiley-VCH GmbH.

## Abstract

L-ascorbic acid 2-phosphate magnesium (APMg) salt is a vitamin C derivative frequently used in cell culture media for research purposes. It is also used as a raw material in the GMP-manufacturing of gene-, cell- and tissue advanced therapy medicinal products (ATMPs). However, quality methods are currently lacking. Therefore, a LC method was developed, based on hydrophilic interaction (HILIC)-ion exchange (IE) mixed-mode liquid chromatography. The final method consisted of an isocratic system with 15 mM $KH_2PO_4$ buffer (pH 2.5 with HCl) acetonitrile (30:70, v/v) mobile phase on a zwitterionic HILIC column, containing an hydrophilic ligand embedded cation-exchange functionality and a surface anion-exchange group. A flow rate of 0.4 mL/min and UV detection at 240 nm was applied. The assay method of APMg was validated, obtaining adequate linearity ($R^2$ = 0.999), precision (RSD of 0.49%) and accuracy (overall recovery of 100.4%). The developed method was successfully applied on five currently marketed products from different suppliers, showing different related substance impurity profiles. Using atomic absorption spectroscopy (AAS), magnesium was found to be bound on the stationary phase, requiring a strong mobile phase to rinse the column. Finally, related impurities were identified using MS/MS and high resolution MS, and found to be ascorbic acid as well as ethyl derivatives, which was further confirmed by NMR.

[*] The author contributed to about 10% to this work.

# 1. Introduction

L-ascorbic acid, also known as vitamin C, is an important vitamin which has various biochemical functions, such as antioxidant effect, enhancement of collagen synthesis in skin fibroblasts and promotion of mesenchymal cells differentiation [1,2]. However, L-ascorbic acid is highly unstable in aqueous conditions which largely limits its full biological application, for example in cell cultures. L-ascorbic acid 2-phosphate magnesium salt (APMg) is a stable derivative of L-ascorbic acid (Fig. 1). The conversion of the 2-OH group to the corresponding phosphate ester prevents the vitamin C molecule to rapidly oxidize into dehydroascorbic acid and further oxidation products. L-ascorbic acid 2-phosphate is highly stable in various aqueous conditions, but it can be easily degraded into L-ascorbic acid in the presence of phosphatases [3]. APMg is frequently used in cell culture media as a L-ascorbic acid surrogate. Next to its slow release antioxidant effect, APMg has additional biochemical functions. It has been shown to increase the growth and replicative lifespan of human corneal endothelial cells, to enhance the survival of human embryonic stem cells and to drive osteogenic differentiation in human adipose stem cells as well as in human mesenchymal stromal cells [4-7]. It is reported that some of these effects are superior to those of ascorbic acid [8].

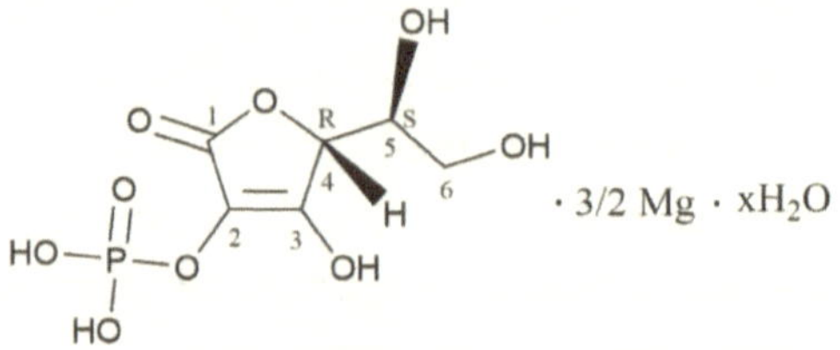

$\cdot\ 3/2\ \mathrm{Mg} \cdot x\mathrm{H_2O}$

**Fig. 1.** The structure of L-ascorbic acid 2-phosphate magnesium (APMg).

Advanced therapy medicinal products (ATMPs), which include gene, cell and tissue engineering medicinal products, offer completely new perspectives for the treatment of severe diseases [9,10]. A new chapter about raw materials for the production of ATMPs was recently adopted in Ph.Eur. and a similar chapter titled "Ancillary materials for cell, gene and tissue-engineered products" was also published in USP [11,12]. The quality of those raw materials used in the production of ATMPs is currently considered a critical aspect in the development of these medicines [13]. Very little is currently known about the critical raw material characteristics that can impact quality and how this quality influences safety and efficacy. APMg is a promising and often-used raw material of ATMPs [14-16]; however, no quality monograph for APMg is currently available in any Pharmacopoeia. The analysis of APMg in cosmetic products is already described, using traditional reversed-phase or ion-pairing liquid chromatography [17-19]. However, retention of APMg in traditional reversed-phase was shown to be insufficient, while ion-pairing generally requires long equilibrium time and dedicated columns and is also incompatible with some detection techniques. Moreover, these analyses did not consider possible related substances. Therefore, an adequate LC method for pharmaceutical GMP quality control of APMg is an urgent need for ATMP developers.

Hydrophilic interaction chromatography (HILIC) can retain polar and ionic solutes that are weakly or not retained on reversed-phase liquid chromatography [20]. The aim of this study was to develop an analytical method using HILIC for APMg. During the analytical development process, the ionization and protonation constants in the mobile phase as well as the behavior of magnesium on the zwitterionic HILIC column were also studied. Hitherto unreported impurities were detected for which their tentative structures are proposed using MS/MS and high resolution MS. Finally, the developed method was validated and applied to commercial samples from different suppliers.

## 2. Materials and methods

### 2.1. Chemicals and reagents

HPLC grade acetonitrile was obtained from Fisher Scientific (Waltham, MA, USA) and ultrapure water of 18.2 M$\Omega$ × cm quality was produced by an Arium pro VF TOC water purification system (Sartorius, Göttingen, Germany). Potassium dihydrogen phosphate, hydrochloric acid and ascorbyl phosphate trisodium salt of analytical grade were supplied by Sigma-Aldrich (St. Louis, MO, USA). Commercial samples of L-ascorbic 2-phosphate magnesium were obtained from Sigma (product code A8960, lot#SLBR3678V; product 1), TCI (product code A2521, lot#R7Q4A-ED; product 2), Discovery fine chemical (product code S22-24/25, lot#75380; product 3), Carbosynth (product code FA76231, lot#1601; product 4) and Santa Cruz Biotechnology (product code SC-228390, lot#I2517; product 5). As no formal official reference standard was currently available, an APMg sample obtained from Sigma-Aldrich with product code

A8960 and lot# SLBS7699 was internally qualified and used as laboratory reference standard. The water content was found to be 21.8% by loss-on-drying and the HPLC purity was found to be above 99.95% using area normalization method.

## 2.2 pH-potentiometric titration

The pH-potentiometric titrations were carried out using an automated Mettler Toledo DL 53 titrator with a Mettler Toledo DG 113-SC pH Electrode. All the solutions used in the titration were prepared in acetonitrile-water mixture (v/v, 70/30). For all the titrations, 30.0 mL of sample solution was titrated with 18.0 mL of 0.05 M NaOH in triplicates at a controlled temperature of 22.0 ± 0.1 °C and ionic strength $I$ = 0.1 mol/L with NaCl. Titrant volumes were added stepwise in aliquots of 0.06 mL.

The protonation constants of the L-ascorbic acid 2-phosphate ligand were determined by pH-metric titrations of 0.01 M ligand prepared in 0.025 M HCl solution. $Mg^{2+}$ solution was prepared at concentration 0.015 M in 0.025 M HCl solution to determine the hydrolysis constants of magnesium. The magnesium coordination complexes with ligand were investigated at ligand-to-magnesium molar ratio 2:3.

Hyperquad 2013® software was used to obtain the protonation constants of the ligand as well as the stability constants of the possible magnesium ligand complexes from the pH-titration results according to the formula (details see Supplementary Information 1) [21]: $\beta_{mlh} = [Mg_mAP_lH_h]\, /\, [Mg]^m[AP]^l[H]^h$ for $m$Mg + $l$AP + $h$H $\rightleftharpoons$ $Mg_mAP_lH_h$, where AP is the L-ascorbic acid 2-phosphate ligand at the fully deprotonated state and m is 0 for the calculation of the protonation constant of ligand. Standard deviations of the stability / protonation constant obtained from titrations (n = 3) were calculated. The autoprotolysis constant of acetonitrile-water mixture (v/v, 70/30) $pK_s$ = 15.88 at 22 °C was used in the equilibrium model [22,23].

## 2.3 HPLC-UV method

Chromatography was performed on an Alliance HPLC system equipped with a Waters 2695 separations module, a Waters 2996 photodiode array detector and Empower 3 Software. An Obelisc N column (3.2 × 150 mm, 5 µm, SIELC Technologies, series: ONNX70UD) was used as stationary phase. The flow rate was 0.4 mL/min and the column temperature was set at 25 °C. The injection volume was

10 µL. UV detection was performed at 240 nm. The mobile phase consisted of a 30/70 v/v mixture of 15 mM $KH_2PO_4$ at pH 2.5 and acetonitrile.

Test and reference solutions for assay purpose were prepared by dissolving 10.0 mg of substance to be examined, respectively reference substance, in water and diluting to 20.0 mL with water. 1.0 mL of the prepared solutions were diluted to 10.0 mL with water for final HPLC injection purposes (assay test solution: 50 µg/mL).

The assay value (content dried substance) of APMg in the sample is calculated as formula 1:

$$\frac{A_x \times m_r \times p}{A_r \times m_x} \times 100\% \tag{1}$$

Where $A_x$ and $A_r$ are the peak area of main component in sample and reference standard; $m_r$ and $m_x$ are the weighted mass of reference standard and sample and $p$ is the purity value of reference standard (*i.e.* 0.782 for our laboratory reference standard).

The impurities were analyzed by dissolving 10 mg of substance to be analyzed in 20.0 mL water (impurity test solution: 500 µg/mL). A reporting threshold of 0.05% was applied and included as a system suitability test for the impurity profile characterization, obtained from a 2000 times dilution of the impurity test solution.

System suitability tests for the APMg assay consisted of the symmetry factor, calculated on the principal peak according to Ph.Eur. (specification: between 0.8 - 1.5), while the repeatability requirement for three reference injections should not be more than 0.62% [24].

## 2.4 Magnesium determination (AAS)

20.0 mg APMg was accurately weighted and dissolved in 20.0 mL water (Mg-stock solution 1). This Mg-stock solution 1 (50 µL) was injected on the HPLC column as described in section 2.3, and the column eluent fractionated in 3 fractions: the eluent before the APMg peak, during the APMg peak and after the APMg peak were collected. Each fraction was diluted to 10.0 mL with mobile phase. The concentration of magnesium in these solutions was determined with AAS (Perkin Elmer,

AAnalyst 200) using 10, 20 and 30 µg/mL APMg reference solution prepared by diluting the Mg-stock solution 1 with mobile phase.

Moreover, after three successive injections of 20 µL 10 mg/mL APMg solution (Mg-stock solution 2), the column was rinsed using 70% 50 mM potassium dihydrogen phosphate and 30% ACN as mobile phase. The eluent was collected from 0-20 min, 20-40 min, 40-60 min, 60-80 min, 80-100 min and these different fractions were diluted to 10.0 mL with rinsing solvent. The concentration of magnesium in these solutions was determined with AAS using 0.5, 5 and 10 µg/mL APMg reference solutions prepared by diluting the Mg-stock solution 2 with rinsing solvent.

## 2.5 HPLC method validation

### 2.5.1 Selectivity solutions

The selectivity of the developed method was confirmed by injecting the blank, ascorbic acid and a crude sample (obtained from Discovery Fine Chemicals, product code S22-24/25). Stress testing was performed by stressing APMg at 0.1 N HCl, 0.1 N NaOH (24 hours, 50 °C) and 0.3% of $H_2O_2$ (1 hour, 50 °C) conditions. APMg was also exposed to daylight for 8 days and UV light for 3 days (photolytic stress) in aqueous solution, according to ICH Guidelines Q1B.

### 2.5.2 Solutions for linearity test

A stock solution containing 0.5 mg/mL APMg reference standard was prepared in water. Different aliquots of this solution were independently diluted in water to obtain five different concentrations, corresponding to 80% (n = 3), 90% (n = 1), 100% (n = 3), 110% (n = 1) and 120% (n = 3) of 50 µg/mL APMg (100%). Calibration curves for peak area versus concentration were plotted and the obtained data were subjected to linear regression analysis.

### 2.5.3 Solutions for limit of detection / quantification (LoD/LoQ)

A 0.1% of 0.5 mg/mL APMg solution was prepared for the determination of LoD/LoQ. The LoD/LoQ was calculated based on the signal-to-noise ratio equaling to 3 and 10, respectively.

## 2.5.4 Solutions for accuracy and repeatability test

Accuracy of the method was tested by performing recovery experiments. APMg solutions were prepared at three levels of 80%, 100% and 120% of 50 µg/mL and each injected in triplicates. The recovery was calculated by comparing the calculated concentration and actual concentration of 100% level. The relative standard deviations (RSD) of triplicate peak areas were calculated for estimation of assay-repeatability. The repeatability and accuracy at related substance level was also performed by injecting triplicates of 0.05%, 0.1% and 0.2% of 0.5 mg/mL APMg solution.

## 2.6 Real sample testing and MS-identification of detected related substances

The anhydrous content of five APMg batches obtained from different suppliers was determined using the developed method. For the identification of the related substances observed in these market samples, the impurity fractions were collected and concentrated using nitrogen gas. The concentrated fractions were further desalted using a prevail organic column (250 × 4.6 mm, 5 µm, Grace, lot#50288608) with mobile phase ACN/water (v/v, 70/30) at flow rate 0.8 mL/min. The other parameters were the same as described in section 2.2. The main peak eluting from this system was collected and the solvent evaporated using nitrogen gas flushing. The residuals were finally dissolved in acetonitrile-water (v/v, 50/50) solvent for the further MS/MS and high-resolution MS analysis.

MS/MS spectra were recorded on a Finnigan LCQ ion trap mass spectrometer with electrospray ionization (ESI) and PC with Xcalibur software version 2.0 by direct infusion with operational settings given in Table 1. The ion-trap MS equipment is a unit mass resolution and low mass accuracy mass spectrometer, with a typical accuracy of 0.1 Da.

High-resolution spectra (accuracy of 0.0001 Da) were recorded on a Waters LCT Premier XE Mass spectrometer in negative mode using leucine enkephalin as calibrant. Samples were infused in water/acetonitrile/formic acid mixture (1:1:0.001 v/v/v) at 100 µL/min. The desolvation gas flow was set to 400 L/hr with a temperature at 200 °C. The cone gas flow was set to 0 L/hr and the source temperature was set to 120 °C. The capillary voltage was set to 2400 V and the cone voltage was set to 40 V. The LCT Premier XE was operated in W mode with a resolution of 11500. The analyser parameters were TOF flight tube 7200 V, reflectron 1800 V, pusher voltage 922 V, MCP 2500 V. Data was acquired in centroid mode.

**Table 1.** Operational parameters for MS/MS data.

| Parameter | ESI⁻ |
|---|---|
| Sheat gas flow rate (arb) | 20 |
| Aux gas flow rate (arb) | 0 |
| Spray voltage (kV) | -4.5 |
| Capillary temperature (°C) | 200.00 |
| Capillary voltage (V) | -18.00 |
| Tube offset (V) | -10.00 |

## 2.7 NMR identification

The $^1$H, $^{13}$C and $^{31}$P NMR experiments were performed on a 600 MHz spectrometer (Bruker Biospin AG, Rheinstetten, Germany) equipped with a 5 mm PABBO BB/19F-1H/D Z-GRD probe at 296 K. Typical acquisition parameters were as follows: $^1$H: 4000 scans (zg30 pulse sequence, baseopt pulse angle 30°); $^{13}$C: 1000 scans (zgpg30 pulse sequence, digital mode, pulse angle 30°); $^{31}$P: 880 scans (zgpg30 pulse sequence, digital mode). 3-(Trimethylsilyl)propionic-2,2,3,3-$d_4$ acid sodium salt (TSP) was used as internal standard for $^1$H NMR. The signal of TSP set at 0 ppm was used as an internal reference for chemical shift ($\delta$) measurement.

Around 15 mg of APMg sample was exactly weighed and mixed with 680 µL $D_2O$ and 20.0 µL of an IS-solution (4.93 mg/mL). The mixture was vortexed until dissolution. 650 µL was then transferred into a 5 mm i.d. NMR sample tube for measurement.

## 3. Results and discussion

### 3.1 pH-potentiometric titration

Using the $pK_a$ values, the ionization degree under selected mobile phase pH can be calculated and further applied to explain the retention behavior of APMg. The typical titration curve of the organic ligand APNa in water-ACN mixture is given in Supplementary Information 2. The $pK_{a1}$, $pK_{a2}$ and $pK_{a3}$ of the $APH_3$ ligand under these conditions were determined as 2.06, 4.40 and 7.17. The species distribution was further calculated as a function of pH and is given in Fig. 2.

The magnesium complex constant in mobile phase condition was also investigated. The formation constant of the aqua-hydroxo complex of magnesium: $[Mg(OH)]^+$, $\log_{10} \beta_{10\text{-}1}$ = -9.49 (m=1, l=0, h=-1) was calculated from the titration of a magnesium chloride solution. Evaluation of the complex formation constants has been carried out for the titrations up to pH 4.0 since then precipitation became visible.

The calculated decimal logarithms of cumulative stability constants are given in Table 2 and the corresponding species distribution curves as a function of pH are given in Fig. 3.

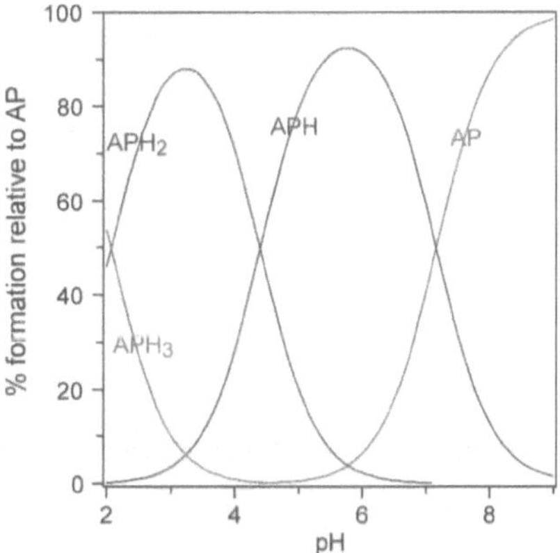


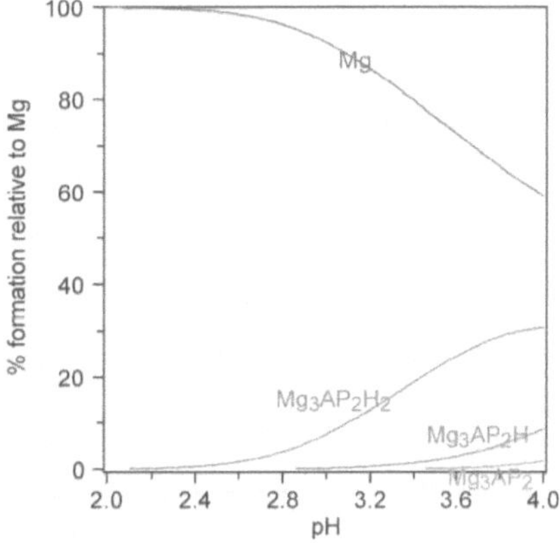


**Fig. 2.** Species distribution curves as a function of pH for the ligand forms: $[APH_3]$, $[APH_2]^-$, $[APH]^{2-}$, $[AP]^{3-}$; $10^{-2}$ M APNa in solvent mixture ACN/water (v/v,70/30).

**Fig. 3.** Species distribution curves for the complexes formed in Mg – AP system at ligand-to-metal molar ratio 2:3 in ACN/water mixture (v/v, 70/30) as a function of pH relative to Mg; $1.5\times10^{-2}$ M $Mg^{2+}$.

**Table 2.** Decimal logarithms of cumulative stability constants $\beta_{mlh}$ = $[Mg_mAP_lH_h]$ / $[Mg]_m[AP]_l[H]_h$ at 22.0 ± 0.1 °C and $I$ = 0.1 M, with standard deviations in parentheses.

| Species | $\log_{10} \beta_{mlh}$ |
| --- | --- |
| $Mg_3AP_2$ | 14.45(11) |
| $Mg_3AP_2H$ | 19.15(6) |
| $Mg_3AP_2H_2$ | 23.70(2) |

## 3.2 Method development

APMg is a polar compound with a charged phosphate group and complexed with magnesium. Traditional reverse-phase LC did not give sufficient retention. An initial column screening was performed and a zwitterionic HILIC column was selected, which has shown its potential for the analysis of polar and charged analytes [20]. This column (Obelisc N), consisting of negative charges near the surface of the stationary phase, a polar – hydrophilic neutral space and positive charges at the end of this space standing in the mobile phase, is a mixed mode column. Electrostatic (ionic) as well as hydrophilic interactions are involved in the interaction of the ascorbylphosphate analyte with this HILIC stationary phase (supporting data see Supplementary Information 3). Two other zwitterionic columns (ZIC-HILIC and ZIC-c HILIC) as well as a pure silica HILIC column (Partisil Silica) were also tried in this study. Only the ZIC-c HILIC column, which has a similar stationary phase structure as the Obelisc N column, showed good retention and peak shape, while the ZIC-HILIC and the Silica HILIC columns did not give reasonable retention, respectively yielded severe tailing.

After the column was selected, the composition of the mobile phase was further adjusted. Acetonitrile, a strongly preferred organic solvent in most HILIC applications, was applied in this study. Different mobile phase additives have also been studied and phosphate buffer was finally selected. When using ammonia formate or ammonia acetate as the mobile phase buffer, a broad tailing peak of APMg was observed (chromatograms see Supplementary Information 4). However, when phosphate buffer was used, the quality of the analyte peak (shape and symmetry) was greatly improved. This observation is consistent with previous findings that severe peak tailing of phosphate compounds was observed when using mobile phase without phosphoric acid or phosphate buffer [25-27]. The peak tailing observed with formate or acetate buffer was supposed to be caused by interaction between the phosphate group of AP and stainless steel in the LC system, while this can be suppressed by introducing phosphate buffer into the mobile phase [25]. The pH of the mobile phase should be below 4 because at higher pH values, precipitation was observed in the pH potentiometric titration of organic ligand / magnesium mixture at mole ratio 2:3. APMg has a maximum absorbance at around 240 nm, making UV detection possible.

Finally, the mobile phase was optimized to be a 30/70 v/v mixture of 15 mM potassium dihydrogen phosphate buffer adjusted to pH 2.5 with HCl solution and acetonitrile. The pH of the applied mobile phase mixture was measured and found to be 3.5. At that pH, most of the organic ligand (around 80%) is at the free ionized state according to the species distribution curve of the possible complexes (Fig. 3), while the predominant species of the free organic ligand is mono-deprotonated (Fig. 2). Thus, APMg is eluting from the column in the form of mono-deprotonated organic ligand, and not as Mg-ligand complexes. This species-derived conclusion was consistent with the observation that the injection of ascorbyl phosphate trisodium salt $APNa_3$ had the same retention time as the magnesium complex APMg.

## 3.3 Magnesium fate on column

To understand the magnesium (from APMg) behavior on the applied column, the fractions which were collected before, during and after the APMg peak were concentrated and analyzed for magnesium content with AAS. Complexed magnesium and ionized magnesium have the same AAS response (details see Supplementary Information 5), allowing to use APMg as a reference substance for the AAS-quantification of magnesium. No magnesium was detected in the collected LC-fractions, indicating that magnesium was retained on the column. According to the species distribution (Fig. 3), approximately 80% of magnesium is in the free ionic form and 20% in the form of the $Mg_3AP_2H^{2+}$ complex under the applied mobile phase condition. A dynamic equilibrium between magnesium and its organic ligand on the one hand and between magnesium and the negative charges of the stationary phase on the other hand is existing. From the AAS results, it can be concluded that under the chromatographic conditions, the binding strength between magnesium and organic ligand is much weaker than that between magnesium and the negative charges of the stationary phase.

To wash magnesium off the column, a mobile phase consisting of 70% 50 mM potassium dihydrogen phosphate and 30% ACN was applied (rinsing phase). The eluent was collected and concentrated for AAS analysis. Magnesium was found in the collected eluent with a recovery of 102.4%. These results proof that magnesium was bound to the stationary phase under the applied assay conditions: the ionic strength of the isocratic mobile phase was too low to wash magnesium off the column. When the ionic strength was increased (rinsing phase), the retained magnesium was eluted from the column. The column in-use stability was proven by 25 consecutive 10 µL-injections of 50 µg/mL APMg solution: no significant difference was observed for retention time as well as peak area among these injections. Even when the column was saturated with magnesium, only a slight increase of retention time (around 0.06 min) was observed for the AP-ligand (details see Supplementary Information 6). However, as a recommendation of Good Chromatographic Practices, it is still recommended to regenerate the column after the APMg analysis with a high ionic strength mobile phase as described above.

## 3.4 Method validation

In order to prove the reliability and applicability of the proposed method, a method validation was performed after the chromatographic conditions have been established. The specificity of the method was confirmed by comparing the chromatograms of blank, ascorbic acid and a crude sample. Stress tests were also performed, however, no degradant peaks were observed. A representative HPLC-overlay chromatogram is given in Fig. 4, in which the impurity peaks are well separated from APMg. Moreover, no impurity peak was found to co-elute with APMg as demonstrated by the DAD peak purity analysis (purity angle 0.040 < purity threshold 0.255).

The linearity between peak area and concentration was obtained for APMg within the range of 80-120% of target concentration (50 µg/mL). Good linearity ($R^2$ = 0.9987) was obtained with a calibration curve of y = (33491±397)x + (24237±20067) going through the origin in 80-120% of target concentration (ANOVA table see Supplementary Information 7). Thus, a one-point-reference method can be used to determine the assay of APMg in an efficient way.

The LoD/LoQ was calculated to be 0.017% and 0.052% of 0.5 mg/mL, respectively, showing that the method was sensitive enough for the determination of related substances at low concentration level.

The precision and accuracy for assay purpose were performed at three levels of 80%, 100% and 120% of 50 µg/mL and the precision as well as accuracy at related substance level were also verified at three levels of 0.05%, 0.1% and 0.2% of 0.5 mg/mL. Three replicates were injected at each level. The RSD% and recovery% were calculated to evaluate the precision and accuracy respectively. The accuracy and precision results are calculated and represented in Table 3, indicating both are good at assay as well as at related substance level.

**Table 3.** Precision and accuracy parameters.

| Concentration(µg/mL) | n[a] | Precision (RSD%)[b] | Accuracy (recovery%)[c] |
|---|---|---|---|
| 40 (80% level) | 3 | 0.486 | 99.93 |
| 50 (100% level) | 3 | 0.459 | 100.40 |
| 60 (120% level) | 3 | 0.217 | 99.74 |
| 0.25 (0.05% level) | 3 | 6.353 | 97.10 |
| 0.5 (0.1% level) | 3 | 2.753 | 96.53 |
| 1 (0.2% level) | 3 | 1.606 | 101.18 |

[a] Number of replicates.

[b] Specification: 2% for active substance, 10% for related substance.

[c] Specification: 98-102% for active substance, 90-110% for related substance.

## 3.5 Structure elucidation of APMg and its related impurities by MS

When applying the developed method to commercial samples, four impurity peaks were found at Rt 2.8, 5.1, 5.6 and 6.7 min, respectively. A typical chromatogram is given in Fig. 4. The peak at Rt 2.8 min was confirmed as ascorbic acid by comparing its retention time to that of the ascorbic acid reference. The impurities at Rt 5.1, 5.6 and 6.7 min were named as Imp1, Imp2 and Imp3, respectively. APMg and the three unknown impurities were characterized by HRMS as well as MS/MS. The HRMS data of those compounds are summarized in Table 4 and the MS/MS spectra are given in Fig. 5.

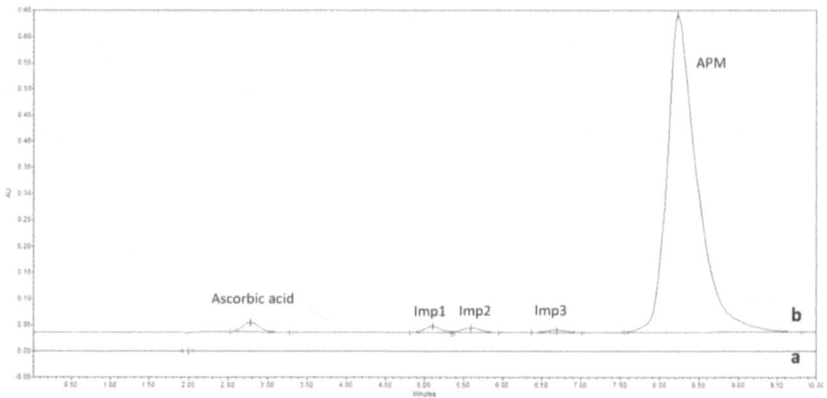


**Fig. 4.** Typical chromatograms of a) blank, b) an APMg sample.

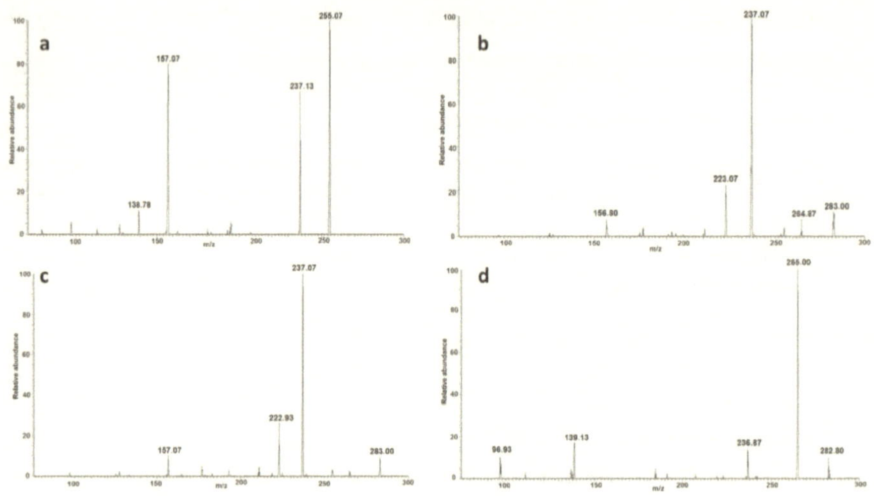

**Fig. 5.** MS/MS spectra of: a) APMg, b) Imp1, c) Imp2, d) Imp3.

**Table 4.** High resolution mass spectral data of APMg and its impurities obtained in negative mode.

| Compound | Ion formula | Found (Da) | Calculated (Da) | Error (mDa) |
|---|---|---|---|---|
| APMg | $C_6H_8O_9P^-$ | 254.9902 | 254.9906 | -0.4 mDa |
| Imp1 | $C_8H_{12}O_9P^-$ | 283.0222 | 283.0219 | 0.3 mDa |
| Imp2 | $C_8H_{12}O_9P^-$ | 283.0215 | 283.0219 | -0.4 mDa |
| Imp3 | $C_8H_{12}O_9P^-$ | 283.0212 | 283.0219 | -0.7 mDa |

### 3.5.1 MS information of APMg

High resolution MS of APMg configured formula [M-H]⁻ was $C_6H_8O_9P$ (experimental mass 254.9902; calculated mass 254.9906, error -0.4 mDa). In the MS/MS spectrum (Figure 5a), the major fragment ion at 237 was a water loss from the parent ion. Another major fragment ion at 157.0 was a $PO_3H$ loss from fragment ion at 237. This loss of phosphate moiety in the form of $HPO_3$ is consistent with previous findings of other organic phosphate compounds [28]. The proposed fragmentation pathway is shown in Figure 6a.

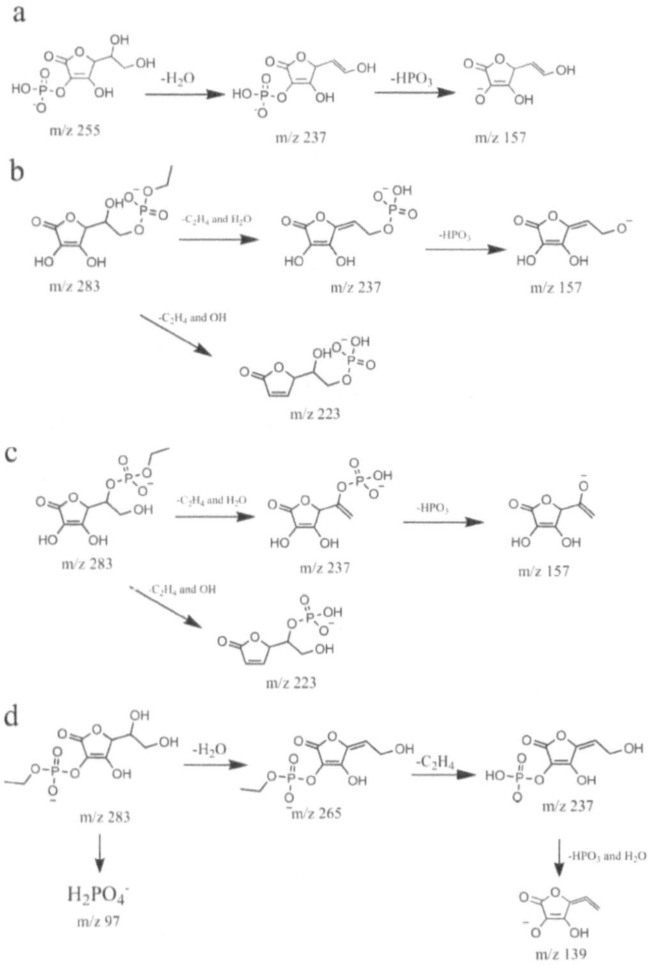

**Fig. 6.** Proposed fragmentation of: a) APMg, b) Imp1, c) Imp2, d) Imp3.

## 3.5.2 MS information of Imp1, Imp2 and Imp3

High resolution MS of Imp1, Imp2 and Imp3 configured formula $[M-H]^-$ was the same $C_8H_{12}O_9P^-$ (Table 4), indicating that these three impurities are isomers. Compared to APMg, these three impurities contain an extra $C_2H_4$ moiety. Phosphorus oxychloride was reported to be used for phosphorylating L-ascorbic acid at $C_2$ in the manufacturing process of APMg [29]. During this process, by-products can be generated when phosphorylation occurred at the two other active hydroxyl groups: $C_5$

and $C_6$ (Fig. 1). Since ethanol was also reported to be used in the manufacturing process, these three impurities can be rationalized as the esterification products from ethanol and phosphate at $C_2$, $C_5$ or $C_6$ of ascorbic acid.

To assign the location of phosphate ester for each impurity, the MS/MS spectra of these three impurities were investigated (Fig. 5b-d). The MS/MS spectra were identical for Imp1 and Imp2, both containing the main fragment ions at m/z 237, 223 and 157. Imp3 showed a different MS/MS fragment profile with main m/z peaks at 265, 237 and 139, revealing a structure difference between Imp3 and the two other impurities. Imp3 could thus be assigned as the $C_2$ enol phosphate ester, while Imp1 and Imp2 have similar structures with the phosphate ester at $C_5$ or $C_6$, respectively. Under the HILIC chromatographic conditions, the most polar compound will generally elute later. Taking into account that primary alcohols are more hydrophilic than secondary alcohols, and neglecting all other interactions, Imp1 is assigned to the secondary alcohol (b in Fig. 6) and Imp2 is assigned to the primary alcohol (c in Fig. 6). The proposed pathways of APMg, Imp1, Imp2, and Imp3 fragmentation are shown in Fig. 6a-d.

## 3.6 Identification of related substances by NMR

In order to further elucidate the structure of the detected impurities, NMR experiments were applied. The atom labelled structure of the impurities were given in Supplementary Information 8 using Imp1 as example, where H-4 represent the protons of methylene groups, H-5 represent the protons of methyl groups, C-7 represent the carbons of methylene groups and C-8 represent the carbons on methyl groups.

The $^1$H NMR spectra of the commercial APMg product containing unknown impurities enlarged in different regions were given in Supplementary Information 9. Besides the APMg signal, a lot of ethyl group signals were also observed from the $^1$H spectrum. With the help of $^{13}$C, $^{31}$P, H-C HSQC, H-C HMBC and H-P HMBC information, different hydrogen signals were carefully assigned (tabulated assignment information as well as the $^{13}$C, $^{31}$P NMR spectra can be found in Supplementary Information 10). Ethanol as well as six ethyl derivatives were detected by NMR in this commercial APMg product.

The structure of Imp1 as proposed by MS was positively confirmed by NMR. The other, multiple impurities observed in NMR were also all ethylated derivatives, consistent with our MS findings. However, the ethyl-isomers were resolved in NMR but not completely in our LC method.

### 3.7 Assay of APMg in commercial samples

Finally, the developed method was applied for the assay determination of APMg products obtained from three different suppliers in the market. Significant quality differences were found between these five commercial products (Table 5), emphasizing the importance of using consistent raw materials in the ATMP production.

**Table 5.** QC results of APMg commercial samples.

| | Product1 | Product2 | Product3 | Product4 | Product5 |
|---|---|---|---|---|---|
| Assay content | 80.55% | 83.67% | 70.59% | 86.15% | 86.38% |
| Related substances | < RT[1] | VitC: 0.10% | VitC: 1.60%<br>Imp1: 1.04%<br>Imp2: 0.88%<br>Imp3: 0.48% | < RT[1] | < RT[1] |

[1]No impurity above reporting threshold (RT of 0.05%) was detected.

## 4. Conclusion

In this paper, a HILIC method for the analysis of APMg was developed, basically validated and applied to commercial products from different suppliers. The chromatographic behavior of magnesium in APMg was studied with the help of AAS analysis and a column regeneration method was proposed based on the results. During the analysis of commercial samples, four impurities were detected and one was confirmed as ascorbic acid using the ascorbic acid reference. The other three unknown impurities were identified as the ethylation products of APMg by MS/MS, HRMS and NMR.

## Conflict of Interest

No conflicts to disclose.

## Acknowledgments

The authors gratefully acknowledge the financial support granted to X.X. by the Ph.D. grant of the China Scholarship Council (CSC) and to M.W. by the Medical University of Łódź (Statute Fund No. 503/3-014-02/503-31-001).

The authors also would like to thank Mr. Izet Karalic for his kind help in HR-MS analysis and Dr. Matthias Grüne and the working group members of Jun. Prof. Dr. Ann-Christin-Pöppler for providing the 600 MHz spectrometer and their qualified advice.

## Appendix A. Supplementary data

Supplementary material related to this article can be found, in the online version, at doi:https//doi.org/10.1016/j.jpba.2018.12.010.

## References

[1] S.R. Pinnell, Regulation of Collagen Biosynthesis by Ascorbic-Acid - a Review. Yale J Biol Med, 58 (1985) 553-559.

[2] D. Chan, S.R. Lamande, W.G. Cole, J.F. Bateman, Regulation of Procollagen Synthesis and Processing during Ascorbate-Induced Extracellular-Matrix Accumulation Invitro. Biochem J, 269 (1990) 175-181.

[3] A. Kokado, H. Arakawa, M. Maeda, New electrochemical assay of alkaline phosphatase using ascorbic acid 2-phosphate and its application to enzyme immunoassay. Anal Chim Acta, 407 (2000) 119-125.

[4] M.K. Furue, J. Na, J.P. Jackson, T. Okamoto, M. Jones, D. Baker, R.I. Hatal, H.D. Moore, J.D. Sato, P.W. Andrews, Heparin promotes the growth of human embryonic stem cells in a defined serum-free medium. P Natl Acad Sci USA, 105 (2008) 13409-13414.

[5] M. Kimoto, N. Shima, M. Yamaguchi, S. Amano, S. Yamagami, Role of Hepatocyte Growth Factor in Promoting the Growth of Human Corneal Endothelial Cells Stimulated by L-Ascorbic Acid 2-Phosphate. Invest Ophth Vis Sci, 53 (2012) 7583-7589.

[6] L. Kyllonen, S. Haimi, B. Mannerstrom, H. Huhtala, K.M. Rajala, H. Skottman, G.K. Sandor, S. Miettinen, Effects of different serum conditions on osteogenic differentiation of human adipose stem cells in vitro. Stem Cell Res Ther, 4 (2013).

[7] X. Fang, H. Murakami, S. Demura, K. Hayashi, H. Matsubara, S. Kato, K. Yoshioka, K. Inoue, T. Ota, K. Shinmura, H. Tsuchiya, A Novel Method to Apply Osteogenic Potential of Adipose Derived Stem Cells in Orthopaedic Surgery. Plos One, 9 (2014).

[8] K. Tsutsumi, H. Fujikawa, T. Kajikawa, M. Takedachi, T. Yamamoto, S. Murakami, Effects of L-ascorbic acid 2-phosphate magnesium salt on the properties of human gingival fibroblasts. J Periodontal Res, 47 (2012) 263-271.

[9] K. Cichutek, Gene and cell therapy in Germany and the EU. J Verbrauch Lebensm, 3 (2008) 73-76.

[10] K.F. Buckland, H. Bobby Gaspar, Gene and cell therapy for children--new medicines, new challenges? Adv Drug Deliv Rev, 73 (2014) 162-169.

[11] Ph. Eur. 9.2, 50212 (01/2017).

[12] General Chapter <1043> Ancillary Materials for Cell, Gene and Tissue Engineered Products. USP 29–NF 24, 1 January 2006.

[13] EMA, Raw materials for the production of cell-based and gene therapy products. symposium report (2013).

[14] J.P. Martins, J.M. Santos, J.M. de Almeida, M.A. Filipe, M.V.T. de Almeida, S.C.P. Almeida, A. Agua-Doce, A. Varela, M. Gilljam, B. Stellan, S. Pohl, K. Dittmar, W. Lindenmaier, E. Alici, L. Graca, P.E. Cruz, H.J. Cruz, R.N. Barcia, Towards an advanced therapy medicinal product based on mesenchymal stromal cells isolated from the umbilical cord tissue: quality and safety data. Stem Cell Res Ther, 5 (2014).

[15] P. Janicki, P. Kasten, K. Kleinschmidt, R. Luginbuehl, W. Richter, Chondrogenic pre-induction of human mesenchymal stem cells on beta-TCP: Enhanced bone quality by endochondral heterotopic bone formation. Acta Biomater, 6 (2010) 3292-3301.

[16] A. Necas, L. Planka, R. Srnec, M. Crha, J. Hlucilova, J. Klima, D. Stary, L. Kren, E. Amler, L. Vojtova, J. Jancar, P. Gal, Quality of Newly Formed Cartilaginous Tissue in Defects of Articular Surface after Transplantation of Mesenchymal Stem Cells in a Composite Scaffold Based on Collagen I with Chitosan Micro- and Nanofibres. Physiol Res, 59 (2010) 605-614.

[17] E. Sottofattori, M. Anzaldi, A. Balbi, G. Tonello, Simultaneous HPLC determination of multiple components in a commercial cosmetic cream. J Pharm Biomed Anal, 18 (1998) 213-217.

[18] Y. Shih, Simultaneous determination of magnesium L-ascorbyl-2-phosphate and kojic acid in cosmetic bleaching products by using a microbore column and ion-pair liquid chromatography. J AOAC Int, 84 (2001) 1045-1049.

[19] A. Semenzato, R. Austria, C. Dallaglio, A. Bettero, High-Performance Liquid-Chromatographic Determination of Ionic Compounds in Cosmetic Emulsions - Application to Magnesium Ascorbyl Phosphate. Journal of Chromatography A, 705 (1995) 385-389.

[20] X.L. Xu, B. Gevaert, N. Bracke, H. Yao, E. Wynendaele, B. De Spiegeleer, Hydrophilic interaction liquid chromatography method development and validation for the assay of HEPES zwitterionic buffer. J Pharm Biomed Anal, 135 (2017) 227-233.

[21] P. Gans, A. Sabatini, A. Vacca, Investigation of equilibria in solution. Determination of equilibrium constants with the HYPERQUAD suite of programs. Talanta, 43 (1996) 1739-1753.

[22] M.A. Herrador, A.G. Gonzalez, Potentiometric titrations in acetonitrile-water mixtures: evaluation of aqueous ionisation constant of ketoprofen. Talanta, 56 (2002) 769-775.

[23] J. Barbosa, V. Sanznebot, Autoprotolysis Constants and Standardization of the Glass-Electrode in Acetonitrile Water Mixtures - Effect of Solvent Composition. Anal Chim Acta, 244 (1991) 183-191.

[24] Ph. Eur. 9.2, 20246 (07/2016).

[25] A. Wakamatsu, K. Morimoto, M. Shimizu, S. Kudoh, A severe peak tailing of phosphate compounds caused by interaction with stainless steel used for liquid chromatography and electrospray mass spectrometry. Journal of Separation Science, 28 (2005) 1823-1830.

[26] G. Shi, J.T. Wu, Y. Li, R. Geleziunas, K. Gallagher, T. Emm, T. Olah, S. Unger, Novel direct detection method for quantitative determination of intracellular nucleoside triphosphates using weak anion exchange liquid chromatography/tandem mass spectrometry. Rapid Commun Mass Sp, 16 (2002) 1092-1099.

[27] J. Zhang, Q.G. Wang, B. Kleintop, T. Raglione, Suppression of peak tailing of phosphate prodrugs in reversed-phase liquid chromatography. J Pharm Biomed Anal, 98 (2014) 247-252.

[28] J.P. DeGnore, J. Qin, Fragmentation of phosphopeptides in an ion trap mass spectrometer. J Am Soc Mass Spectr, 9 (1998) 1175-1188.

[29] Y.K.Y. Ishimura, Method for producing L-ascorbic acid 2-phosphates, 5110951, 1992.

## 5. Supplementary Information

*SI 1*

In Hyperquad 2013, the stability constants refinement is based on minimization of non-linear least-squares sum [1] The refinement process involves calculating the "shift" which is added to the log $\beta$ value but limited to about 2.5 log units. The refinement is protected against shift values over a number of refinement cycles that are more than this amount. In the case of the diverging refinement, the parameter shift vector is reduced in length. This allowed to find a set of parameters giving a lower sum of squares. After 10 attempts not reducing the sum of the squares, the refinement is completed. Refinement progress is over-written each time a refinement is made. The details of each iteration are stored until convergence is reached and stored [1].

The objective function $U = \sum_{i=1}^{m} W_i \, r_i^2$ was used to check the goodness of fit, where $m$ is the number of experimental points, $W_i$ is the weight and $r$ is a residual, equaling to the difference between observed and calculated values of pH. The value of the normalized sum of squared residuals, $\sigma = U/(m\text{-}n)$ was compared with chi-squared test of randomness at a number of degrees of freedom equal to $m\text{-}n$ ($n$ is the number of refined parameters).

Different models with varies complexes ($Mg_mAP_lH_h$) were proposed to Hyperquad 2013® software. The complexes with obtained stability constants which are impossible or have very large errors will be rejected from the system. The result of the refinement is considered unsatisfactory. With standard deviations on log $\beta$ of about 0.1 or less, the 95% confidence limits range about two standard deviations about the refined parameter value. The model selection process and the standard deviation calculation are associated with an error in the electrode measurement. Too low concentrations of species (do not reach 10% of the total metal/ligand concentration) make it difficult to establish the stability constants. Also when the $\beta$ value of one species is highly correlated with the $\beta$ value of another species they will have the same high pH effect [2].

***SI 2***

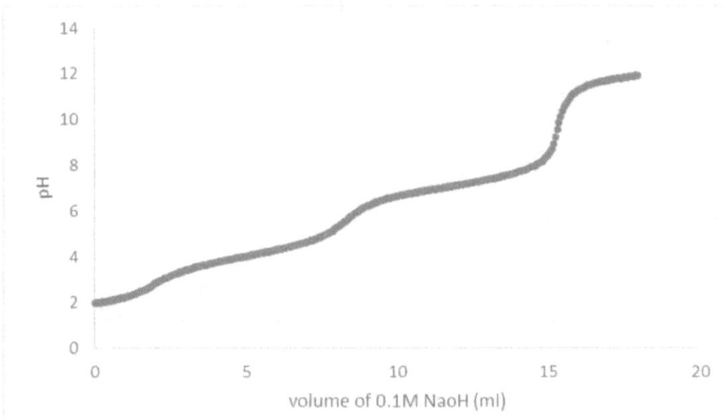

**Fig. S1.** The typical titration curve of 0.01 M organic ligand given in relation of volume of 0.1 M NaOH solution and pH.

***SI 3***

The retention behavior of APMg was investigated under different mobile phase conditions (chromatograms see Fig. S2-4). With a change in buffer strength from 10 mM to 20 mM, the retention time of the AP ligand decreased from 8.38 min to 5.56 min (see Fig. S2). This sharp decrease in AP ligand retention time is an indication for a significant role of ionic interaction in the retention mechanism of AP ligand. Additionally, with a decrease of ACN content from 70% to 65% in the mobile phase, the retention time of AP ligand decreased from 8.38 min to 7.91 min. This observation is consistent with a hydrophilic behavior.

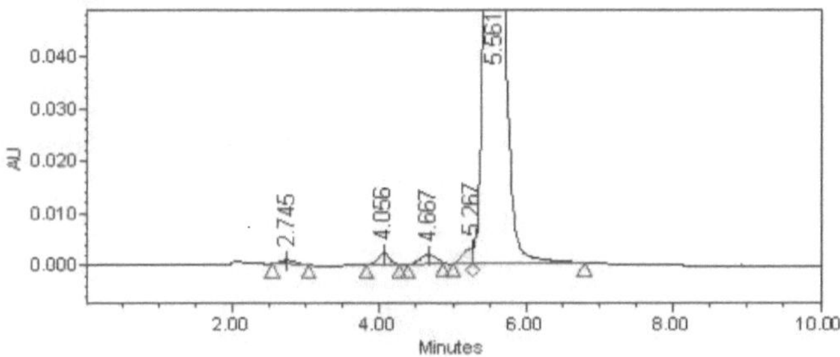

**Fig. S2.** The typical chromatogram of APMg product at mobile phase condition: 70:30 (V/V) ACN/ 20 mM $KH_2PO_4$ with 0.1% $H_3PO_4$ (main peak at 5.56 min).

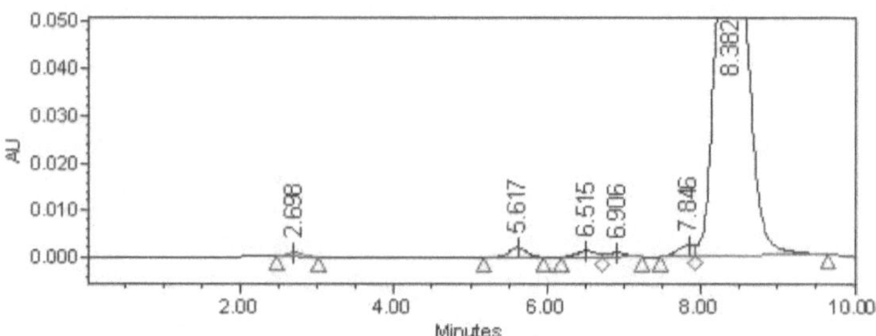

**Fig. S3.** Chromatogram of APMg product at mobile phase condition: 70:30 (V/V) ACN/ 10 mM $KH_2PO_4$ with 0.1% $H_3PO_4$ (main peak at 8.38 min).

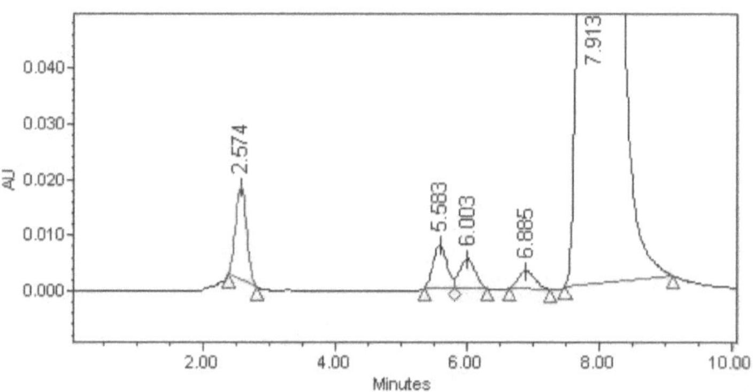

**Fig. S4**. Chromatogram of APMg product at mobile phase condition: 65:35 (V/V) ACN/ 10 mM $KH_2PO_4$ with 0.1% $H_3PO_4$ (main peak at 7.91 min).

*SI 4*

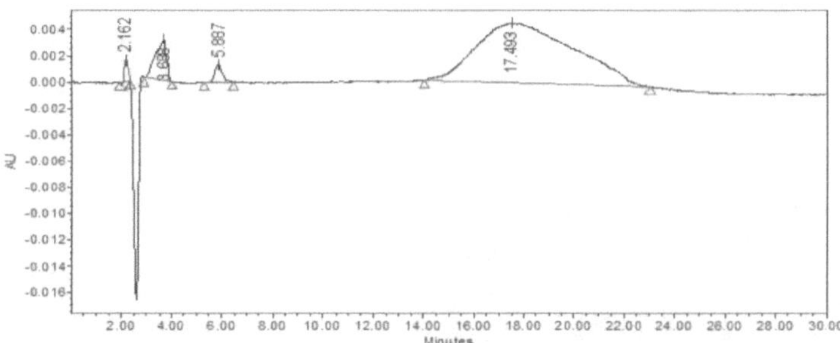

**Fig. S5.** Chromatogram of APMg when using mobile phase consisted of a 30/70 v/v mixture of 15 mM ammonia formate at pH 2.5 and acetonitrile. The other conditions are the same as described in section 2.3.

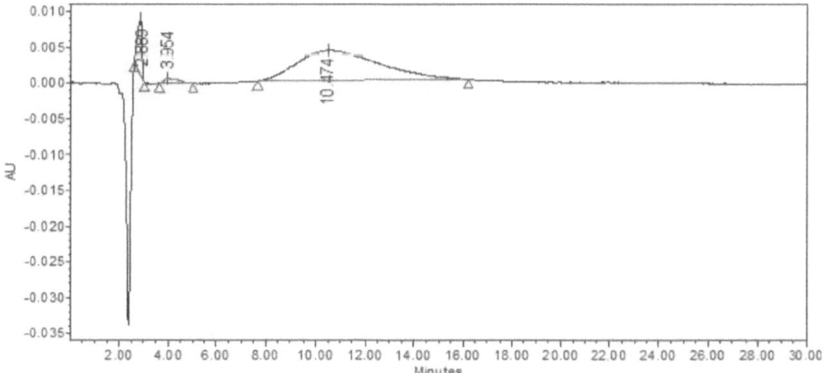

**Fig. S6.** Chromatogram of APMg when using mobile phase consisted of a 30/70 v/v mixture of 50 mM ammonia formate at pH 2.5 and acetonitrile. The other conditions are the same as described in section 2.3.

## *SI 5*

The magnesium reference solutions at 0.03, 0.05, 0.1, 0.15 and 0.2 ppm prepared from $MgSO_4 \cdot 7H_2O$ were analyzed using AAS. The absorbance of each reference solution was recorded and given in Table S1.

**Table S1.** AAS results of magnesium reference solutions.

| Reference concentration/ppm | Absorbance |
| --- | --- |
| 0.03 | 0.044 |
| 0.03 | 0.044 |
| 0.03 | 0.044 |
| 0.05 | 0.063 |
| 0.05 | 0.063 |
| 0.05 | 0.063 |
| 0.1 | 0.124 |
| 0.1 | 0.125 |
| 0.1 | 0.125 |
| 0.15 | 0.177 |
| 0.15 | 0.178 |
| 0.15 | 0.179 |
| 0.2 | 0.239 |
| 0.2 | 0.238 |
| 0.2 | 0.239 |

The plot of absorbance versus concentration was made in the concentration range 0.03 - 0.2 ppm and given in Fig. S7, with R square 0.9993.

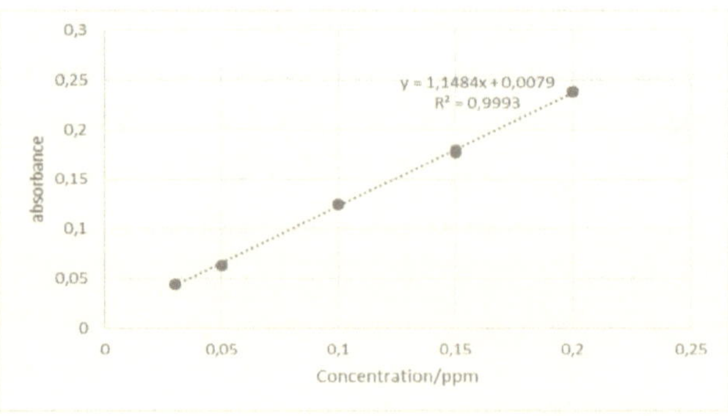


**Fig. S7.** Linearity curve of magnesium reference solutions in concentration range 0.03 - 0.2 ppm.

The APMg (Sigma, product code A8960, lot#SLBR3678V) solutions at *l.c* concentration 0.03, 0.05, 0.1, 0.15 and 0.2 ppm were analyzed using AAS. The absorbance of each solution was recorded and given in Table S2. The concentration of solution at *l.c.* 0.05 ppm was calculated using the calibration curve of magnesium reference ($y = 1.1484x + 0.0079$). The other points were updated according to this point and given in a new column. The absorbance versus the corrected concentration was plotted and given in Fig. S8. Both curves show good linearity in the selected range. The slope of both curves was slightly different from that of magnesium reference.

**Table S2.** AAS linearity results of APMg solution.

| *l.c* Mg concentration/ppm | Corrected concentration/ppm | Absorbance |
|---|---|---|
| 0.03 | 0.026 | 0.039 |
| 0.03 | 0.026 | 0.04 |
| 0.03 | 0.026 | 0.04 |
| 0.05 | 0.043 | 0.057 |
| 0.05 | 0.043 | 0.057 |
| 0.05 | 0.041 | 0.055 |
| 0.1 | 0.086 | 0.109 |
| 0.1 | 0.086 | 0.109 |
| 0.1 | 0.086 | 0.109 |
| 0.15 | 0.128 | 0.155 |
| 0.15 | 0.128 | 0.156 |
| 0.15 | 0.128 | 0.156 |
| 0.2 | 0.171 | 0.205 |
| 0.2 | 0.171 | 0.207 |
| 0.2 | 0.171 | 0.206 |

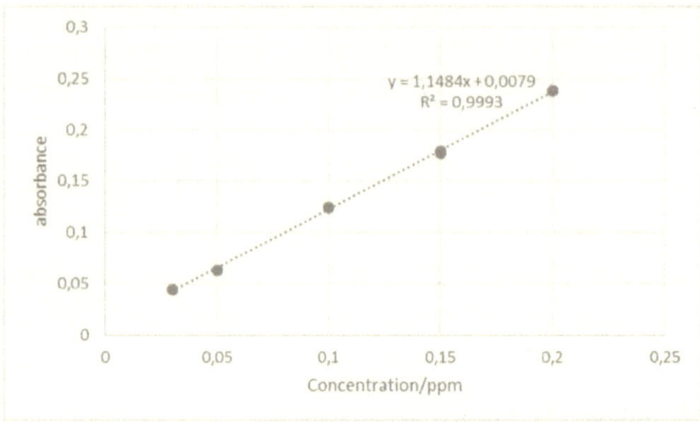


**Fig. S8.** Linearity curve of APMg solutions in magnesium concentration range around 0.03 - 0.2 ppm.

### *SI 6*

Twenty-five (25) injections of 50 µg/mL APMg were performed to mimic a reasonable routine analysis, and the target peak of the AP ligand was evaluated. The RSD value of retention times as well as of the peak areas of these 25 injections were experimentally determined and found to be 0.10% and 0.31%, respectively, indicating a good in-use stability of the developed method. A Mg saturated column was prepared with the following steps:

1) The column was rinsed with 70% of 50 mM $KH_2PO_4$ (brought at pH 2.5 by hydrochloric acid) and 30% of ACN to remove the retained magnesium on the column.
2) The column was equilibrated with the applied mobile phase: 30% 15 mM $KH_2PO_4$ (brought at pH 2.5 by hydrochloric acid) and 70% ACN.
3) Switch mobile phase to magnesium containing mobile phase (2.4 µg/mL Mg). The eluents were collected in fractions of 15 minutes (6 mL), and analyzed with AAS. The magnesium containing mobile phase was prepared by dissolving 20.3 mg $MgCl_2·6H_2O$ in 20.0 mL mobile phase (same as step 2). 4.0 mL was further diluted to 200.0 mL with the same mobile phase. Calculation see below:

$$C = 20.3 \; mg \; \times \frac{24.3}{203.3} \times \frac{1}{20 \; mL} \times \frac{4 \; mL}{200 \; mL} = 0.0024 \text{ mg/mL} = 2.4 \text{ µg/mL}$$

The eluents from step 3 were collected every 15 minutes per tube and the magnesium content was analyzed by AAS. Results were summarized in Table S3. No magnesium was found until the collection 23, indicating that the column under the applied HILIC condition was saturated with Mg after 345 minutes (23×15). Thus, the magnesium capacity of the column was calculated as below:

Capacity of $Mg^{2+}$ = 345 min × 0.4 mL/min × 2.4 µg/mL = 331 µg $Mg^{2+}$

**Table S3.** Magnesium in the collected elution detected by AAS.

| Sample | Absorbance |
| --- | --- |
| Blank | 0.001 |
| Mg containing MF (2.4 µg/mL) reference | 0.321 |
| Collection 1 | 0.002 |
| Collection 2 | 0.001 |
| Collection 3 | 0.003 |
| Collection 21 | 0.003 |
| Collection 22 | 0.004 |
| Collection 23 | 0.087 |
| Collection 24 | 0.325 |
| Collection 25 | 0.322 |
| Collection 26 | 0.319 |

The retention time and peak area of trisodium ascorbyl phosphate salt (APNa), APMg and HEPES on Mg-free and Mg-saturated column under the developed HPLC method was compared (Table S4).

Retained $Mg^{2+}$ can slightly increase the retention time of APNa and APMg. However, a more obvious decrease in retention time was found for HEPES. There is no positive charge center in the AP ligand, thus, the block of negative charge of the stationary phase is indeed expected to have no influence on the ligand retention. The retained magnesium may increase the water layer, leading to a slightly increase of retention time of the ligand. For HEPES, a zwitterionic compound which has a positive charge center, the blocked negative ends of the stationary phase by $Mg^{2+}$ can weaken the interaction between HEPES and the stationary phase, leading to an earlier elution.

**Table S4.** Peak parameter difference between Mg free and Mg saturated column.

| Parameter | Sample (n=3) | Mg free column | Mg saturated column |
|---|---|---|---|
| Retention time | APNa | 8.24±0.01 | 8.34±0.01 |
| | APMg | 8.25±0.01 | 8.31±0.01 |
| | HEPES | 10.92±0.06 | 10.23±0.05 |
| Peak area | APNa | 1846686±7137 | 1848708±7482 |
| | APMg | 1626027±2545 | 1626399±1557 |
| | HEPES | 1104972±5136 | 1098569±6051 |

*SI 7*

**Table S5.** ANOVA results for APMg.

| | df | SS | MS | F | Significance F | |
|---|---|---|---|---|---|---|
| Regression | 1 | 7.291E+11 | 7.291E+11 | 7128.317 | 2.324E-14 | |
| Residual | 9 | 9.205 E+11 | 1.023E+8 | | | |
| Total | 10 | 7.300E+11 | | | | |
| | *Coefficients* | *Standard Error* | *t Stat* | *P-value* | *Lower 95%* | *Upper 95%* |
| Intercept | 24236.517 | 20066.696 | 1.208 | 0.258 | -21157.503 | 69630.538 |
| X Variable 1 | 33490.877 | 396.673 | 84.429 | 2.324E-14 | 32593.539 | 34388.214 |

*SI 8*

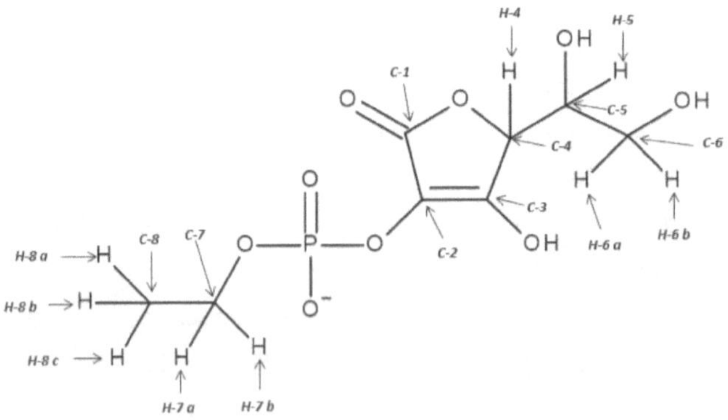

**Fig. S9.** Atom labelled Impurity 1. H-7 a,b represent the protons of methylene groups, H-8 a,b,c the protons of methyl groups. C-7 represent the carbons of methylene groups, C-8 the carbons on methyl groups.

*SI 9*

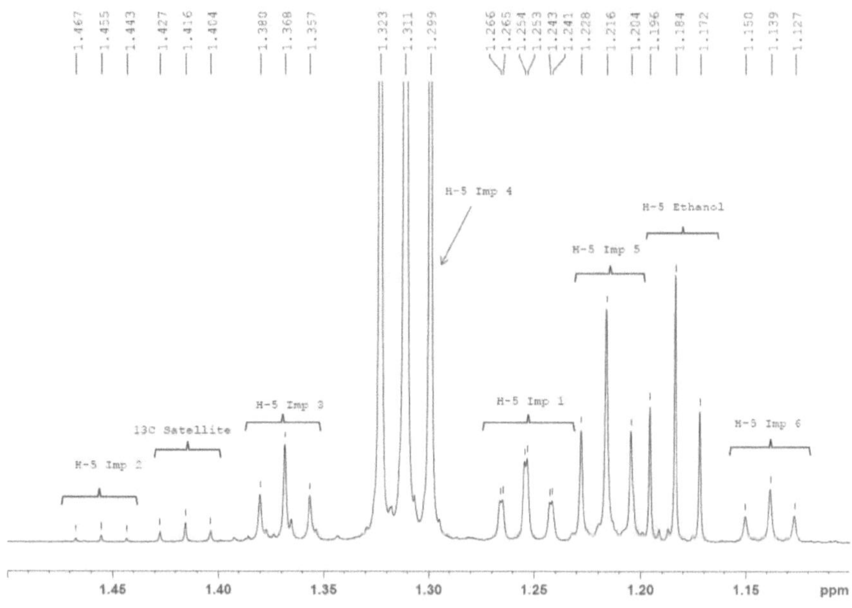

**Fig. S10a.** ¹H NMR spectrum of APMg product in the region 1.1 - 1.5 ppm. Imp 1 - Imp 6 are considered being ethylated derivatives of APMg.

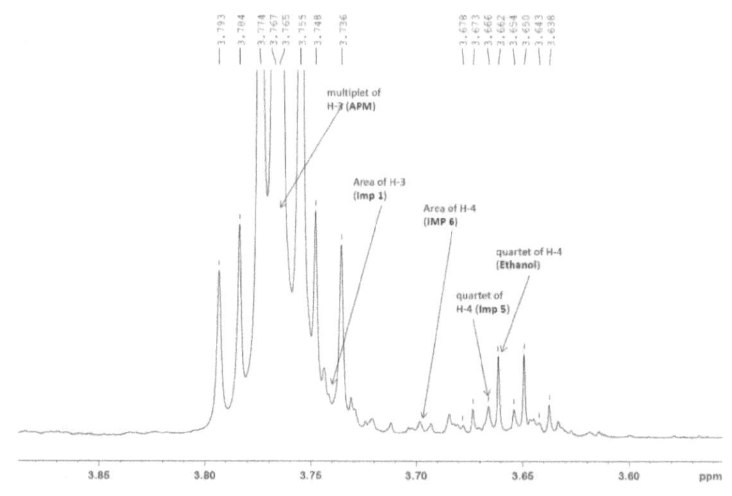

**Fig. S10b.** ¹H NMR spectrum of APMg product in the region 3.55 - 3.90 ppm.

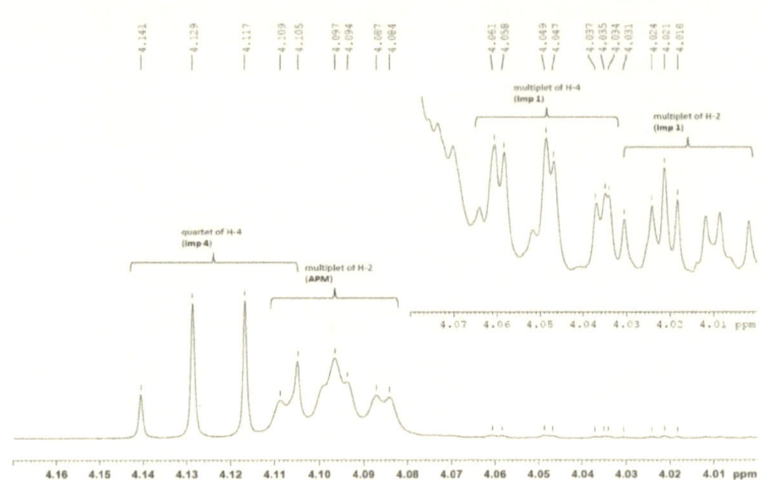

**Fig. S10c.** $^1$H NMR spectrum of APMg product in the region 3.9 - 4.2 ppm.

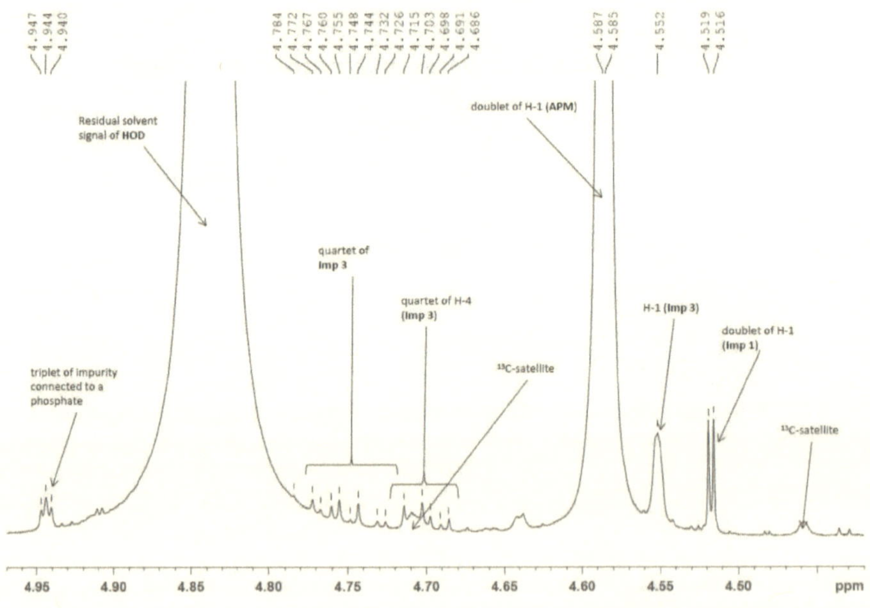

**Fig. S10d.** $^1$H NMR spectrum of APMg product in the region 4.45 - 4.98 ppm.

***SI 10***

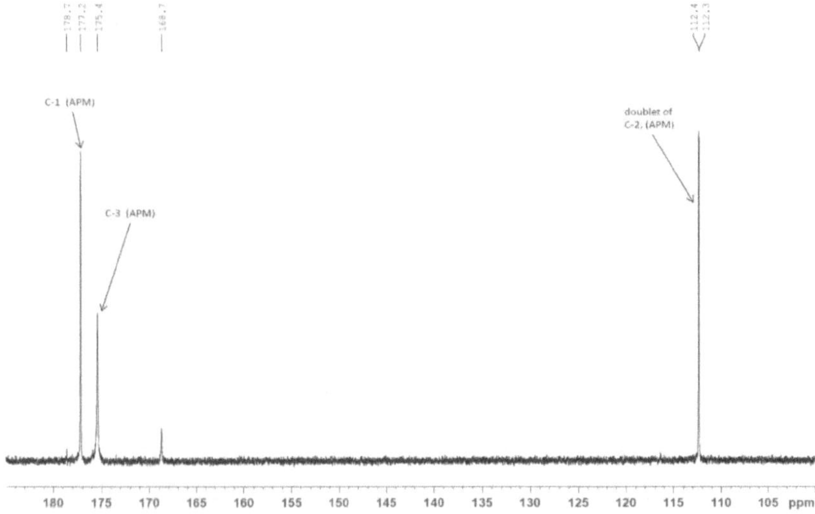

**Fig. S11.** $^{13}$C NMR spectrum (600 MHz) of APMg product in the region 100 - 180 ppm.

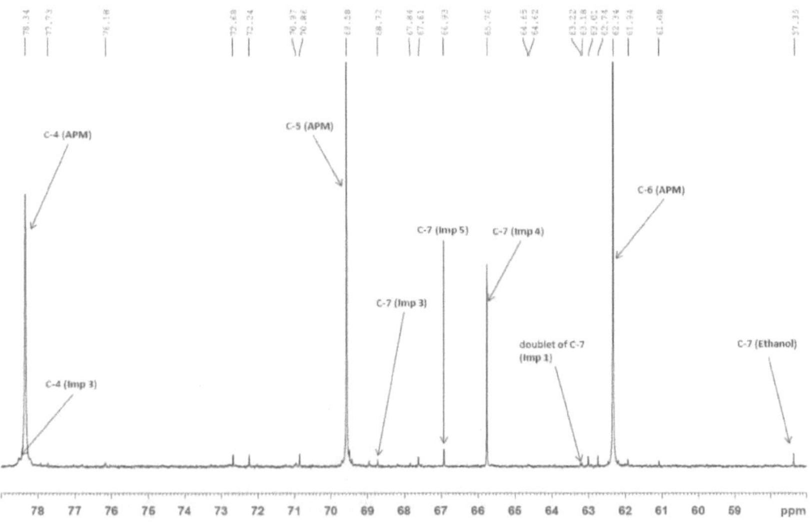

**Fig. S12.** $^{13}$C NMR spectrum (600 MHz) of APMg product in the region 57 - 79 ppm.

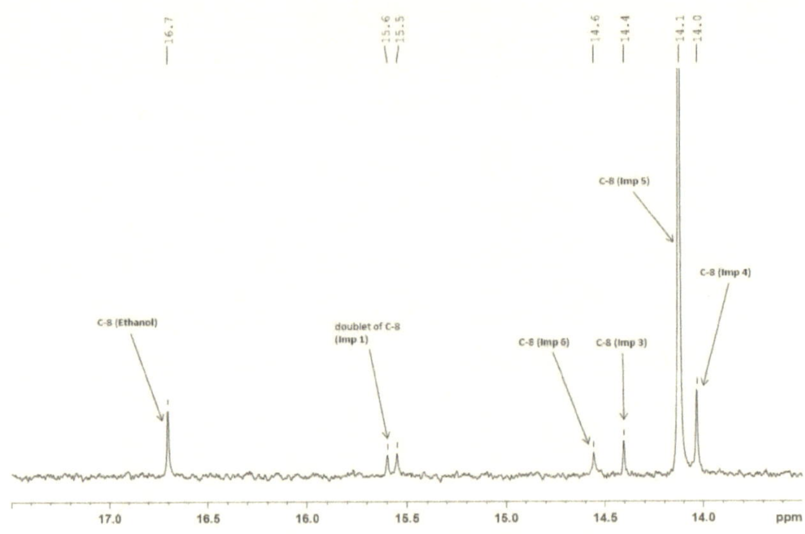

**Fig. S13.** $^{13}$C NMR spectrum (600 MHz) of APMg product in the region 13 - 18 ppm.

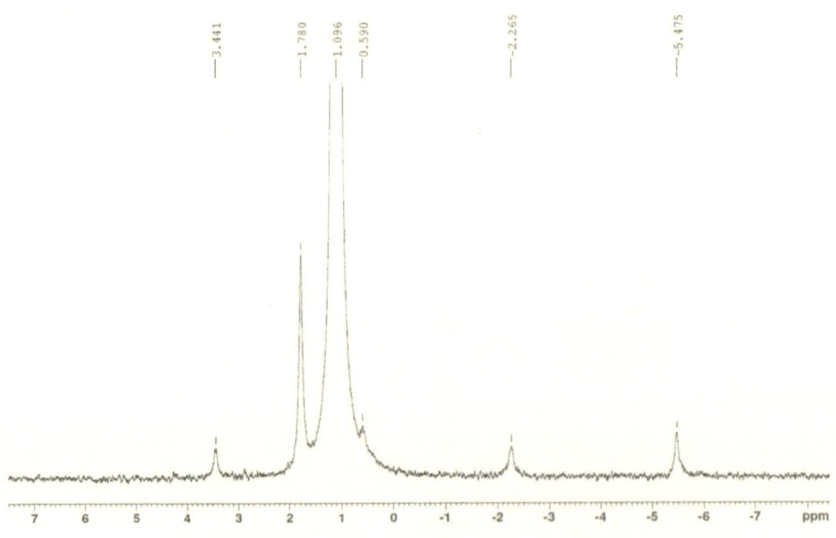

**Fig. S14.** $^{31}$P NMR spectrum (600 MHz) of A2PMg product.

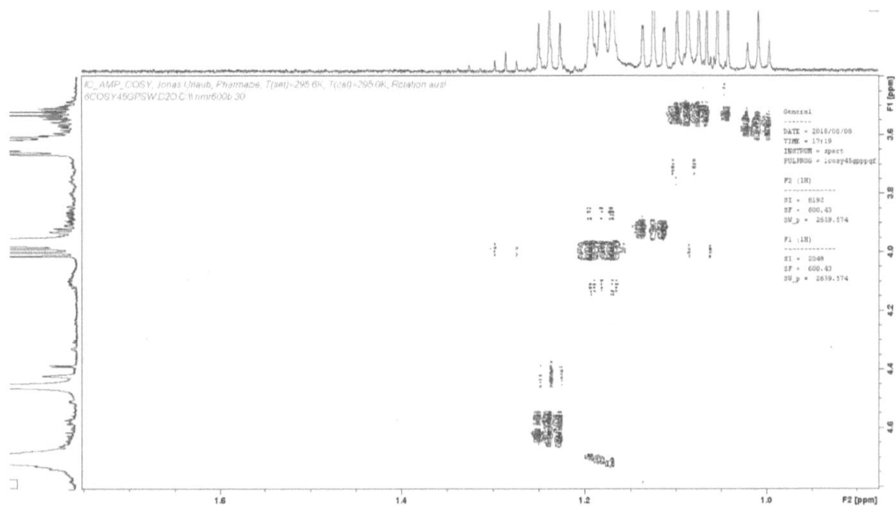

**Fig. S15.** COSY of APMg fine chemicals (600 MHz) - The $^{13}$C satellites are marked with circles.

**Table S6.** $^{13}$C NMR data. s: singulet; d: doublet; t: triplet; q: quartet; m: multiplet.

| signal $^{13}$C NMR<br>δ (ppm) | cross signals H,C - HSQC<br>δ (ppm) $^1$H | cross signals H,C-HMBC<br>δ (ppm) $^1$H | interpretation |
|---|---|---|---|
| 178.7 | - | 4.06 (t) | - |
| 177.2 | - | 4.59 (d) | C-1 (APMg) |
| 175.4 | - | 4.59 (t); 4.10 (m) | C-3 (APMg) |
| 168.7 | - | - | - |
| 112.3 (d, 5.5 Hz) | - | 4.59 (d) | C-2 (APMg) |
| 78.7 | 4.55 (s) | | C-4 (Imp 3) |
| 78.3 | 4.59 (s) | 3.76 (m) | C-4 (APMg) |
| 77.7 | 3.87 (s) | - | - |
| 76.2 | 4.94 (s) | - | - |
| 72.7 | 4.00 (s) | 3.63 (m) | - |
| 72.2 | 4.06 (s) | 3.63 (m) | - |
| 71 | 3.93 (s) | - | - |
| 70.9 | 3.71 (d) | 3.66 (m) | - |
| 69.6 | 4.10 (s) | 3.76 (m) | C-5 (APMg) |
| 68.7 | 4.71 (s) | 1.37 (m) | C-7 (Imp 3) |
| 67.8 | 3.70 (s) | 1.14 (m) | C-7 (Imp 6) |
| 67.6 | 4.23 (s) | - | - |
| 66.9 | 3.66 (s) | 1.22 (m) | C-7 (Imp 5) |
| 65.8 | 4.12 (s) | 1.31 (m) | C-7 (Imp 4) |
| 64.6 (d) | 3.98 (s) | - | - |
| 63.2 (d) | 4.05 (s) | 1.25 (m) | C-7 (Imp 1) |
| 63.0 | 3.64 (s) | - | - |
| 62.7 | 3.77 (s) | - | - |
| 62.3 | 3.76 (s) | 4.59 (d); 4.10 (s) | C-6 (APMg) |
| 61.9 | 3.8 – 3.7 (s) | - | - |
| 61.08 | 3.78 (s) | - | - |
| 57.4 | 3.66 (s) | 1.18 (m) | C-7 (Ethanol) |
| 16.7 | 1.18 (s) | 3.66 (q) | C-8 (Ethanol) |
| 15.6 (d, 5.8 Hz) | 1.25 (s) | - | C-8 (Imp 1) |
| 14.6 | 1.14 (s) | - | C-8 (Imp 6) |
| 14.4 | 1.37 (s) | - | C-8 (Imp 3) |
| 14.1 | 1.31 (s) | 4.12 (q) | C-8 (Imp 4) |
| 14 | 1.22 (s) | 3.66 (s) | C-8 (Imp 5) |
| -3.0 | 0 | 0 | TSP |

**Table S7.** $^{31}$P NMR data of APMg product.

| signal $^{31}$P NMR<br>$\delta$ (ppm) $^{31}$P | cross signals<br>H,P - HMBC<br>$\delta$ (ppm) $^{1}$H | interpretation |
|---|---|---|
| 4.18 (no $^{31}$P-signal) | 3.8 (quintett);<br>3.50 (s) | - |
| 3.445 (m) | 3.97 (m); 3.83 (d) | - |
| 3.29 (no $^{31}$P-signal) | 4.55 | - |
| 2.90 (no $^{31}$P-Signal) | 3.84 (t); 1.22 (t) | - |
| 1.82 | -- | - |
| 1.053 | 4.59 (m), 4.55 (d) | P (APMg) |
| 0.66 | 3.93 (t) | - |
| 0.57 | 4.94 (d) | - |
| 0.45 (no $^{31}$P-signal) | 3.97 (t) | - |
| -2.32 | 4.55 (d); 4.05 (m);<br>1.25 (m) | P (Imp 1) |
| -3.31 | 4.08 (quartett);<br>4.98 (s), 1.28 (s) | - |
| -9.76 | 4.02 (t) | - |

# References


[1] P. Gans, A. Sabatini, A. Vacca, Investigation of equilibria in solution. Determination of equilibrium constants with The HYPERQUAD suite of programs, Talanta, 43 (1996) 1739-1753.

[2] P.V. Hyperquad 2013, User's Guide. Protonic Software.

9 783384 273451